Sick and Tired of Being Sick and Tired

ch. 5-6

University of Pennsylvania Press
Studies in Health, Illness, and Caregiving
Joan E. Lynaugh, General Editor

A complete list of books in this series appears at the end of this volume.

Sick and Tired of Being Sick and Tired

Black Women's Health Activism in America, 1890–1950

Susan L. Smith

University of Pennsylvania Press
Philadelphia

Portions of Chapter 5 appeared in an earlier form in "White Nurses, Black Midwives, and Public Health in Mississippi, 1920–1950," *Nursing History Review* 2 (1994): 29–49. Reprinted by permission.

Library of Congress Cataloging-in-Publication Data
Smith, Susan Lynn, 1960–
    Sick and tired of being sick and tired : black women's health activism in America,
1890–1950 / Susan L. Smith.
        p.   cm. — (Studies in health, illness, and caregiving)
    Includes bibliographical references and index.
    ISBN 0-8122-3237-2 (alk. paper). — ISBN 0-8122-1449-8 (pbk. : alk. paper)
    1. Afro-American women health reformers — Southern States — History.
2. Afro-Americans — Medical care — Southern States — History.   3. Health care reform —
Southern States — History.   4. Public health — Southern States — History.   I. Title.
II. Series.
RA448.5.N4S65   1995
362.1′089′96073 — dc20   95-11310
                                                                        CIP

Contents

Figures

Acknowledgments

This book began in 1985 as a seminar paper in a graduate course at the University of Wisconsin-Madison on "Women in American Reform Movements 1890–1920," with Linda Gordon and visiting historian Ellen Du-Bois. That research paper grew into a master's thesis on black club women under Gerda Lerner in 1986 and a dissertation on black women's public health work under Judith Walzer Leavitt in 1991. Now it is finally a book. It has been a long, hard process. However, I had the privilege of working with an outstanding community of scholars in the Women's History Program who helped me in numerous ways. In particular, I extend my deepest gratitude to Andrea Friedman, Linda Gordon, Judith Walzer Leavitt, Gerda Lerner, Leslie Reagan, and Leslie Schwalm for all I have learned from them. Each woman has profoundly influenced my thinking and therefore this book.

The book had another beginning in 1985 in the Women's Studies Program at the University of Wisconsin-Madison. That year Nancy Worcester and Mariamne Whatley hired me to be a teaching assistant for the introductory course on women's health. My three years associated with that course not only helped pay the rent but shaped the direction of my research. Both Nancy and Mariamne taught me much about women's health and the women's health movement, which prompted my examination of black women's health activism in the past. Judy Leavitt's superb course on the history of women and health gave me the opportunity to pursue my new interest. At the end of my graduate career I had the chance to attend Vanessa Northington Gamble's course on the history of race, American medicine, and public health, the first such course taught in the United States. These courses in women's studies, women's history, and the history of medicine have helped to clarify my own research agenda.

Wisconsin has proved to be a rich reservoir of friendships and scholarly support over the years. I would like to thank the following people for their vital assistance, including comments on earlier drafts of this material and kind words at just the right moment: Karen Booth, Jeanne Boydston, Kathleen Brown, Suzanne Desan, Eileen Findlay, Maureen Fitzgerald, Joyce

Follet, Jennifer Frost, Maureen Galitski, Vanessa Northington Gamble, Nancy Isenberg, Carl Kaestle, Marie Laberge, Anne Lewis, Laura McEnaney, Nellie McKay, Leisa Meyer, Lisa Peck, Mary Peckham, Doris Stormoen, and Janet Wright.

Since moving in 1991 to Canada, where universal health care is more or less a reality, I have found a new network of support. I thank my colleagues at the University of Alberta, especially Laurie Adkin, Linda Bridges, Lesley Cormack, Susan Hamilton, David Marples, Patricia Prestwich, and Frances Swyripa, for helping me to make Canada my home.

Finally, several other scholars have offered valuable critical assessments of some or all of this material at key points in the creation of this book. In particular I want to thank Barbara Brodie, Darlene Clark Hine, Nancy Tomes, and Molly Ladd-Taylor for their astute observations, and Robynne Healey and Amrita Chakrabarti Myers for excellent research assistance. I also want to thank the audiences who responded with warmth and keen interest to various presentations of my research throughout the late 1980s and early 1990s at the following conferences: the Southern Conference on the History of Women, the Berkshire Conference on the History of Women, the American Association for the History of Medicine Conference, the First International Conference for the History of Nursing, the Smithsonian Institution Lecture Series on Black Health, the University of Wisconsin System Women's Studies Conference, the conference on Black Health: Historical Perspectives and Current Issues, the Midwest Graduate Feminist Studies Conference, and the National Women's Studies Association Conference.

It is customary to conclude the acknowledgments with thanks to one's family, but it seems more appropriate to do so now. This book would have never reached completion, at least in this century, without the incredible support of my partner Donald Macnab. A psychologist by training, he knew just the right words to say when self-doubt clouded my confidence and yet one more task threatened to preempt my writing. I will forever remember his loving refrain: "get the book done!" The birth of my daughter Caitlin, under the skillful guidance of midwives Sandy Pullin and Susan James, and my two other lively children, Erin and Andreas, provided additional incentives to finally finish, while the care of Marie Hughes made it possible. My first family gave me further encouragement, especially my parents Lori and Bob Smith, as well as my brothers Jerry and Larry, my aunts Norma and Carole, my grandmother Charlotte, and my best friends Karen SheltonBaker and Pamela Beals. In each of their own special ways, they contributed to the completion of this book. I only regret that my mother, who died in 1994, did not live long enough to see the final product.

In an era of dwindling resources for students, I would like to acknowledge the financial support that I received as a graduate student from my family and granting agencies. Without that aid, completing a dissertation would have been a far more difficult task. I received financial assistance for research and writing from several sources at the University of Wisconsin-Madison, including a KNAPP Women's History Fellowship Grant, Graduate School Domestic Travel Fellowship, and Maurice L. Richardson Fellowship from the History of Medicine Department at the University of Wisconsin Medical School. The Woodrow Wilson National Fellowship Foundation awarded me a Women's Studies Research Grant and a very generous Rural Policy Fellowship. I also received travel grants from the Central Research Fund at the University of Alberta.

In conclusion, I extend my appreciation to the archivists and individuals who made my research trips profitable and enjoyable experiences. In Washington, D.C., special thanks to Bettye Collier-Thomas, formerly of the Bethune Museum and Archives; Esme Bhan of Moorland-Spingarn Research Center at Howard University; and Aloha South at the National Archives. I also thank Daniel T. Williams and Helen Mahone at Tuskegee University, and Anne Lipscomb at the Mississippi Department of Archives and History in Jackson. Finally, special thanks to the following individuals for agreeing to share their memories with me: Dr. Paul Cornely, Jessie Guzman, Edna Roberts, and the late Mabel Staupers and Dr. W. Montague Cobb. They helped me keep my focus on the human side of health reform.

Introduction: African Americans, Gender, and Public Health in the South

Black health activism in the United States emerged at a time when the American welfare state was expanding and black rights were decreasing. From 1890 to 1950, a period of legalized segregation, many African Americans saw their struggle for improved health conditions as part of a political agenda for black rights, especially the right to equal access to government resources. Although it was difficult for a group with little influence on government to affect public policy, black activists struggled to draw federal attention to black health issues. They tried to make the health needs of black America a legitimate political concern for the nation. With great caution they entered the debate on the role of the state in the care of its citizens.

Black health reform was gendered to the extent that men held most of the formal leadership positions and women did most of the grassroots organizing. Much like the black civil rights movement of the 1950s and 1960s, "men led, but women organized."[1] Black men played an important role in the black health movement as doctors, ministers, journalists, businessmen, and educators. Yet, men's leadership often came and went, while women's grassroots activity persisted.[2]

Indeed, there is a continuous, unbroken line of black women's health activism since at least the 1890s. Black female professionals and community leaders formed the backbone of the black health movement and were central to the founding and maintenance of black public health projects. They implemented health reform measures at the local level and thus translated health policy into health programs. Furthermore, black women were the primary targets of black public health work because of their influence on the physical and moral health of their families.

The history of black women's health activism demonstrates the ongoing contributions of laywomen to public health work. Despite the increasing involvement of white, and some black, health professionals and government officials in health and welfare work after 1930, much of the history of black health work is the history of layworkers. Laywomen played a key role because segregation severely limited the number of black medical experts; they made health programs available to a larger proportion of their communities than doctors and nurses could ever hope to reach. Black public health work was carried out by midwives, teachers, home demonstration agents, sorority and club women, nurses, and a few dentists and physicians.[3]

In addition to gender, class influenced the shape of black health reform. Class differences among African Americans affected the motivations for and consequences of health projects. There is little agreement among historians on how best to define class status among black Americans because it was so fluid, and racism ensured that even affluent African Americans enjoyed few class privileges within white society. However, by 1910 about 3 percent of the black population, some 300,000 African Americans, had obtained educational training, a degree of economic security, and careers in business or various professions, factors that influenced their middle-class status. Early in this century, tens of thousands of middle-class black activists, "race men" and "race women," struggled to improve the living and working conditions of African Americans. Although they critiqued the impact of racism on health, they occasionally verged on victim-blaming when they stressed changes in individual behavior as the solution to improved black health.[4]

Members of the black middle class faced a dilemma imposed by American racism in how best to provide adequate social welfare services within a segregated system. They encountered contradictory experiences of privilege relative to the black poor but powerlessness in the face of institutionalized racism, with their leadership repeatedly circumscribed.[5] Class tensions and competing interests existed among African Americans, as in most populations, yet shared frustration with racism sometimes led to strong bonds between the black middle class and the poor. This connection at times minimized the distance between helper and helped.

Yet the black poor were not mere silent partners in the quest for health reform, even if the historical records make their activities far more difficult to document.[6] Indeed, despite the low expectations of black and white health officials, poor people's attendance at health clinics and participation in clean-up campaigns attest to their efforts to improve their health. The history of the public health work of midwives illustrates some of the informal, day-to-day public health work carried out by poor rural women.

This book, then, explores the gender, class, and political dynamics of one phase of the history of the black struggle for improved health. The book emerges at the intersection of women's history, African-American history, and the history of medicine. Following recent trends in work on the welfare state, it attempts to move beyond depictions of African Americans only as recipients of aid or victims of neglect.[7] Instead it highlights the ways in which black health activists attempted to create public health programs and influence public policy at every opportunity. Although their efforts were not always successful, they carried out a concerted campaign to address black health needs. Recognizing the vital contributions of African-American women to the history of public health reveals how and why public health work succeeded and where it failed to reach underserved Americans over the last century.

This story of black women's health activism addresses the growing body of scholarship on the welfare state and on the civil rights movement that documents the lines of continuity in twentieth-century social reform. Increasingly, scholars in women's history have emphasized the links between women's social welfare work in the Progressive Era and women's efforts to shape public policy in the New Deal era.[8] Meanwhile, scholars of the modern civil rights movement have identified twentieth-century black protest activities as part of an ongoing black freedom movement.[9] The history of black women's health activism shows that the lines of continuity stretch from the Progressive Era to the New Deal and on into the civil rights era.

Black Health Needs and Public Health Work in the South

Historical literature on public health in the United States has grown rapidly, but enormous gaps remain. The historiography of American health reform generally leaves out both African Americans and women, thereby making black women's reform efforts doubly invisible.[10] Furthermore, much of the history of public health has focused on the growing cities of the North, Midwest, and South, ignoring the rural context even though the majority of white Americans lived in rural areas until 1920 and the majority of black Americans did so until World War II. Even today nearly one-fourth of the American population is rural.[11]

Historians date the start of organized public health work in the South to the 1870s, although there were some activities earlier in the nineteenth century. Southern public health officials focused on urban epidemics during the nineteenth century and increasingly turned their attention to rural health conditions in the early twentieth century. The South remained a predominantly rural region well into the twentieth century because of the slower pace of industrialization.

Public health work in the southeastern United States was influenced by slaveholding, race relations, one-crop economies, climate and geography, and a self-defined sense of a uniquely southern way of life.[12] The New South that emerged from defeat in the Civil War began as white Southerners regained control of local and state governments at the end of Reconstruction in the late 1870s. Former slaves faced inequality in all areas of public welfare, including the justice system, housing, education, and health. By 1890 segregation existed in law as well as in custom.[13]

Racial politics has had a powerful impact on the development of public health in the South. The long history of slavery in the region, the continued presence of a large black population, and the tradition of white supremacy shaped public health policy. Most notably, white determination to maintain social, economic, and political power over African Americans despite the end of slavery fueled resistance to any public welfare programs that might inadvertently benefit black people. At the same time, a key theme in public health during the nineteenth and early twentieth centuries was the fear that sickness among black people could spread to white people, suggesting the need for some public health measures directed at African Americans. African Americans were well aware of this tension in white supremacist ideology between a reluctance to alter power relations and a fear of black illness, and black activists attempted to exploit it to their benefit when campaigning for government programs.

A few historians have begun to analyze the ways racism and segregation restricted black access to health services and social welfare institutions in the past. Edward Beardsley, in particular, has demonstrated the neglect of and outright denial of health services to African Americans in the twentieth-century South.[14] Poverty and discrimination limited opportunities for health services, and thereby increased health needs. The paucity of material about the history of black people's health status and their efforts to improve health conditions is startling. A narrative history of African Americans in medicine, published in 1967 by Herbert Morais, is still unmatched. A few historians have demonstrated the impact of racism on black health but with little comment on how African Americans responded to oppression.[15]

Currently, the history of organized public health efforts in the South can be divided into roughly three periods: (1) the Civil War to 1890, when epidemics prompted the establishment of southern state boards of health;

(2) 1890 to 1915, when private foundations played a major role in sponsoring southern public health campaigns; and (3) 1915 to 1950, when two world wars and the Great Depression led to the expansion of federal government authority over public health. Historians have shown that wars and epidemics had a great impact on health consciousness in the South and across the nation.[16] Of equal importance was the effect of racism, a continuous theme within these stages of historical development.

The Legacy of Slavery and Yellow Fever: Public Health from the Civil War to 1890

White Southerners expressed concern with sanitation and adequate health before the Civil War, but on a private level rather than through any systematic, statewide focus on public health. Yellow fever and, to a lesser extent, cholera prompted public health efforts in urban areas during the antebellum era, but only to a limited degree.[17] Of greater interest to southern slaveholders was the potential threat of epidemics in slave quarters, which they saw as a matter of public health.[18]

Economic interests and the desire for a healthy labor force, as well as the fear that disease could spread to their own families, directly affected slaveowners' concern for the health of black slaves. Often any benefits that black people derived during epidemics were the result of white fears of disease transmission. Owners disposed of wastes around the slave quarters to help control disease. Ill slaves found themselves isolated, sometimes in plantation "hospitals," to prevent the spread of sickness. Despite the wishes of slaves who preferred to treat themselves, slaveholders forced slaves to receive medical care from owners, slave nurses, and, as a last resort, physicians.[19]

In antebellum America the dominant belief among white Southerners was that innate racial differences between black and white people created black and white health disparities and fitted black people to be slaves. Many believed that if black people became sick it was because of an inherently weaker constitution rather than a result of unhealthy living and working conditions. Meanwhile, some physicians argued that African Americans were more resistant then white people to certain diseases, such as yellow fever and malaria, and therefore were better suited to field labor.[20]

Following the Civil War, there is much evidence to suggest that the white South had little concern for freedmen and freedwomen, including their health needs. Concerns about race relations and political and economic reconstruction preoccupied black and white Southerners. Such concerns were evident during epidemics and struggles between white planters and freedpeople over the provision of health services in labor contracts. Plantation owners no longer felt responsible for the health of black workers, and many southern physicians simply refused to treat black people. In general, medical aid and relief, which was in great demand after the war, was less available to black people than to white.[21] Southern provisions of private and public charity, available to many white refugees following the war, were denied to black refugees, while public services available in white sections of town were not extended to black sections. For example, when smallpox struck towns after the war, city governments often simply ignored the disease among black people. In places like Richmond, Virginia most local hospitals refused to care for black people, and when they did treat African Americans they placed them in segregated wards in the least comfortable parts of the facility. In one Atlanta hospital, which received substantial city funding, officials crowded black patients into an annex off the kitchen.[22]

Some white Americans pointed to high morbidity and mortality rates among African Americans as evidence of black racial inferiority and of the benefits slavery had provided. In 1881 the head of the Louisiana State Board of Health reported that in New Orleans the black mortality rate had increased to four times higher than the white rate. Contemporary accounts claimed that some 25 percent of the black population in the city died from poor health after the Civil War. A Montgomery, Alabama newspaper reported on the tragic incident of a black woman who died after giving birth in an old dump cart, only to have the surviving infant eaten by hogs. The newspaper offered the story as evidence of the consequences of the demise of slavery.[23]

The establishment of the Freedmen's Bureau, with its medical division, marked a milestone in the development of federal responsibility for public health. Indeed, historians of the welfare state would do well to note that the first federal welfare measure occurs here in the nineteenth century.[24] The bureau, created by Congress in 1865, stepped in with an underfunded and understaffed medical division to provide some aid to former slaves, even though intended as only a temporary measure. Despite the objections of southern municipal authorities, from 1865 to 1869 the Freedmen's Bureau provided health care to at least some African Americans through the establishment of hospitals, dispensaries, and home-visitation programs. Bureau staff vaccinated black people against smallpox, and in Louisiana the Freed-men's Bureau attempted to stop the spread of a cholera epidemic by inspecting black homes and communities.[25]

As the New South emerged, fighting yellow fever became the priority of public health officials. The needs of industry and commerce influenced public health policy when the 1867 outbreak of yellow fever in New Orleans created a panic in business activity throughout the South. Symptoms of yellow fever included headache, delirium, fever, and "black vomit," the result of blood from internal hemorrhaging. Southern state boards of health developed in the 1870s and 1880s, including Alabama in 1875 and Mississippi in 1877, specifically for the purpose of controlling yellow fever and curbing its impact on southern commerce. Southern state boards of health emphasized quarantine to curb epidemics, while northern state boards of health focused on sanitation activities to control endemic diseases.[26]

The southern yellow fever epidemic of 1878, a widespread outbreak that was particularly costly in lives and dollars, demonstrates how epidemics shaped southern health consciousness. Not only did this epidemic increase civic interest in public health, but it also led to demands from some Southerners for federal assistance, ultimately resulting in the establishment of the National Board of Health. The board existed from 1879 to 1883 as a federal agency in charge of quarantine.[27]

The 1878 yellow fever epidemic illustrates the impact of southern racial ideology and race relations on public health. When yellow fever struck a town, the wealthy white inhabitants left, abandoning the city and its epidemic to the poor, many of whom were black. For example, when the 1878 epidemic struck New Orleans, panic caused 40,000 of the 211,000 inhabitants to leave. Three out of four white people left the city, leaving behind most African Americans, who accounted for 70 percent of the remaining residents. The epidemic even led Memphis, Tennessee to hire its first black police officers because of the shortage of white personnel. Morbidity and mortality reports of the epidemic began to alter white perceptions of the impact of the disease on African Americans. So many black people contracted the disease and died that white beliefs about black immunity were shaken. Part of the explanation for the increased visibility of black ill-health was the increased reporting of black morbidity in the late nineteenth century.[28]

Although yellow fever epidemics resulted in the establishment of state boards of health, racial politics and economic troubles constrained southern health reform efforts in the post-Civil War years. White southern fears of black progress and racial equality significantly slowed the funding and development of southern public health campaigns.

"Racial Degeneration" and Northern Interference: Public Health from 1890 to World War I

Ideas about racial difference and black inferiority held sway during the so-called Progressive Era from 1890 to World War I. Frederick L. Hoffman, a health statistician for the Prudential Life Insurance Company, played a prominent role in promoting such views. In Hoffman's 1896 publication *Race Traits and Tendencies of the American Negro*, he built on the concept of "survival of the fittest," drawn from social Darwinism, to argue that black people were an inferior species headed for extinction because they were no longer "sheltered" slaves. Hoffman placed particular emphasis on the idea of the physical and moral deterioration of black people due to sexual immorality. His views illustrated accepted medical knowledge, thinly veiled by white fears about black sexuality and the existence of a large, free black population.[29]

In 1906 the national black leader W. E. B. Du Bois challenged this bleak forecast and countered arguments of inherent black inferiority in *The Health Physique of the Negro American*, proceedings drawn from an Atlanta conference on black health. The conference findings pointed to the impact of environmental and social conditions on black morbidity and mortality rates. Commenting on the higher black rates, Du Bois noted that "the present differences in mortality seem to be sufficiently explained by conditions of life."[30]

The debate over black physical decline took place during the Progressive Era, a period marked by the growth of a black middle class, a white backlash against African-American progress, and a corresponding increase in black activism. It was a time of escalating violence by white against black Americans, including an increase in lynchings, the legal assault on black communities through the disenfranchisement of black men, and the entrenchment of segregation through the policy of "separate but equal." Many African Americans responded by forming national organizations to combat racism and by leaving the South.[31]

Historians have paid little attention to the impact of such racial politics on early twentieth-century southern public health work. Instead they have focused mostly on the role of northern philanthropic foundations, such as the Rockefeller Foundation, and the federal government in sponsoring southern health campaigns to combat diseases such as hookworm and pellagra.[32] These "southern" diseases brought unflattering national attention to the South during this period. Influenced by the science of bacteriology or germ theory of disease, health officials sought to uncover the causative agents of diseases.

Some white Southerners interpreted northern interest in southern diseases as insulting outside interference. Pellagra, a vitamin deficiency disease that was fairly common in the United States in the nineteenth century, was "discovered" in the South in 1906 when an epidemic struck the black inmates of the Mount Vernon Insane Hospital in Alabama. Symptoms of pellagra included red and scaly skin, stomach disorders, diarrhea, and depression. Both private foundations and the federal government assisted with studies of pellagra. The United States Public Health Service (USPHS) conducted investigations of the disease, and two wealthy northern philanthropists donated $15,000 to study pellagra. Joseph Goldberger of the USPHS conducted research showing that poor southern diet was a prime cause, and he connected diet to the cash-crop southern economic system. Many Southerners resented the stigma of poverty implied by Goldberger's theory of dietary deficiency.[33]

The hookworm eradication campaign from 1910 to 1915, sponsored with one million dollars from the Rockefeller Foundation, added to the perceived assault on southern pride. Hookworms are blood-sucking parasites that enter between the toes of bare feet and live in the intestines, where female hookworms produce eggs that pass out in the feces and hatch in the soil. The hookworm eradication program called for the introduction of sanitary privies or toilets and the wearing of shoes. Some Southerners suspected that depictions of the South as worm-infested was just a way for the Rockefellers to make money by selling shoes to frightened residents. Southern hostility to health and education campaigns by northern foundations was rooted in the Reconstruction era, when resentment of northern interference was at its height.[34]

The Rockefeller Hookworm Campaign did provide direct benefits to underfunded, understaffed, and legally powerless state public health systems. The campaign, which began at the prodding of scientist Charles Stiles at the United States Department of Agriculture, encouraged the creation of local health departments in rural communities throughout the South. In

Mississippi, where health work had long been minimal due to limited state government funding, the Rockefeller Foundation provided money to set up dispensaries in every county in order to provide free examinations and treatment for the disease. Indeed, the Rockefeller Foundation left behind a network of state and local public health agencies.[35]

Contemporaries generally believed that diseases such as hookworm and pellagra affected black and white Southerners in different ways. Historians have repeated these observations without satisfactorily analyzing how or why white Southerners identified such differences. For example, black people supposedly had a lower incidence of pellagra, yet a researcher for the USPHS during the 1910s found that more black than white people died from the disease. Health officials in Mississippi, which kept complete records of its pellagra epidemic, discovered in a 1913 study that black people were just as susceptible to pellagra as white people. The study suggested that the similarity had not been noticed before because black cases had not been counted.[36] Historians also have portrayed black people as less susceptible than white people to hookworm infection. Yet the Rockefeller Foundation performed hookworm eradication work in black communities, even though campaign organizers did not hire black doctors to work with them.[37]

By the early twentieth century the federal government and northern philanthropic foundations were assisting with the development of an institutional base for public health activity in the South. Yet southern health officials continued to neglect the needs of black Americans, except to point to morbidity and mortality figures as evidence of "racial degeneration." Instead, the impetus for rural and urban black public health work came mostly from African Americans.

Federal Authority and the USPHS: Public Health from 1915 to 1950

By World War I health officials acknowledged that African Americans would not become extinct, but they continued to point to racial disparities in health as a sign of black inferiority. Consistently throughout the twentieth century black morbidity and mortality rates were higher than corresponding white rates. For example, in 1900 the black death rate was 25 per 1,000 people, while the white rate was 17 per 1,000, and although the black rate dropped in 1930 to 14 per 1,000, it was still considerably higher than the white rate of 10. In addition, although black and white life expectancy increased over the course of the twentieth century, a gap remained with white rates always higher than black.[38] While some white health officials explained these differences in terms of racial inferiority, black health activists pointed to the influence of socioeconomic factors.

The USPHS expanded southern public health activities, as two world wars and the Great Depression profoundly increased federal authority over public health in the United States. In 1902 President Theodore Roosevelt changed the name of the Marine Hospital Service, founded in 1798 to assist seamen, to the Public Health and Marine Hospital Service in order to acknowledge its expanding activities. In 1912 the institution became the United States Public Health Service, reflecting its exclusive concern with national health issues.[39]

Federally sponsored public health work was wide-ranging. During World War I the USPHS led a major campaign against venereal disease in order to safeguard the health of military recruits. It revived health campaigns against syphilis during the 1930s and 1940s.[40] The Maternity and Infancy Protection Act of 1921, known as the Sheppard-Towner Act, provided federal matching grants to the states. Administered through the federal Children's Bureau throughout the 1920s, the act provided financial support for maternal and child health programs.[41] In the 1930s New Deal legislation attempted to aid national recovery through such health and welfare measures as the 1935 Social Security Act. Reluctant to commit funding to public health measures, southern legislators had to be convinced that the South paid too high a price for its diseased population.[42] Ultimately the federal government rescued the southern health care system and provided the first government health reform measures to benefit African Americans.[43]

However, part of the indigenous roots of public health activity in the twentieth-century South arose from the work of African Americans. Even the limited federal health activity for African Americans during the 1930s rested on a foundation of black health programs put into place by black people well before the New Deal. Indeed, black self-help has been a strong, permanent component of black community life. African Americans were not resigned to ill health; throughout the nation they sought out solutions to sickness in their communities. A more complex history of public health will emerge as historians take into account the health activities of African

Americans whose struggles changed the contours of the southern health landscape.[44] Furthermore, increasing black migration out of the South made black health a national, not just a southern, concern.[45]

*   *   *

This book is the first full-scale effort to examine the health reform initiatives created by African Americans themselves. As I learned from the historian Gerda Lerner, the historical sources are there if one but looks in the right places. Over and over again in my research on the history of black women's health activism, I was struck by the vastness of black history records, many of which lay deteriorating and unprocessed. In official government records at the state and federal level, especially the records of the USPHS, the Children's Bureau, and the U.S. Department of Agriculture, housed at the National Archives in Washington, D.C., I found evidence of how African Americans responded to the inadequate provision of health services. The Library of Congress Manuscript Division, the Bethune Museum and Archives, and the Mississippi Department of Archives and History contain key materials on black health. I analyzed incredibly rich resources at two historically black colleges, Tuskegee University and Howard University, including manuscript collections of national black organizations and individuals active in the movement. Finally, I benefited from reading transcripts of many black women's oral histories and conducting interviews with several black and white activists and health professionals. Such personal sources greatly enriched my understanding of the historical records. Without such material it is difficult to hear the voices of those who make history outside of the limelight.

The first section of this book traces the development of a twentieth-century black health movement. Although I focus on black women's health activism in the South, the first three chapters include discussion of black health campaigns elsewhere because of the widespread activity of the black health movement. The story begins with an analysis of the informal health activities of organized black club women who laid the foundation for the black health movement beginning in the 1890s (Chapter 1). Next I examine the racial and gender politics behind the health education campaign of the National Negro Health Movement, with its annual National Negro Health Week. Black women's health activities can best be understood through comparison to men's; hence much of this discussion focuses on the public health work of male leaders (Chapters 2 and 3). Booker T. Washington launched this nationwide health education program shortly before his death in 1915 in order to call national attention to the pressing need for better health among African Americans. The annual National Negro Health Week activities promoted clean-up campaigns, health education programs, and medical examinations. The era of the National Negro Health Movement, which spanned from 1915 to 1950, marked a complex transition period between the separate black health organizing efforts of the early twentieth century and the integration efforts of the post-World War II period.

In the second section I investigate the implementation of health policy by discussing case studies of black women's public health work in the rural South. These three chapters explore health reform in Alabama and Mississippi, both predominantly rural states with large black populations. They provide an in-depth analysis of the administration of health programs at the local level, where women played a prominent role. As one examines the health education programs of the extension workers with the Tuskegee Movable School in Alabama (Chapter 4) or the public health work of midwives (Chapter 5) and sorority women (Chapter 6) in Mississippi, one realizes that women were the vital links to black communities. Even the Tuskegee Syphilis Study in Alabama (Chapter 4) depended on a black nurse to mediate between the government doctors and the subjects of the experiment. Yet, as these case studies demonstrate, public health work had both progressive and oppressive consequences.

This work shows that middle-class black activists tried to shape government policy by injecting concern for black health into the southern, and national, public health agenda. National Negro Health Week, the Tuskegee Movable School, and the Alpha Kappa Alpha Mississippi Health Project were all demonstration programs that sought to convince governments at the state and federal level to address the needs of black America. Even the black professionals associated with the infamous Tuskegee Syphilis Study believed the study would eventually increase black access to government resources.

This book concludes with some observations on the ways in which black women's tradition of community organizing for health and social welfare continued after 1950. Health issues were, and continue to be, a major focus of black women's political activity, as witnessed most recently in the National Black Women's Health Project, which took the famous words of Fannie Lou Hamer as its slogan. Hamer, the youngest of twenty children born to sharecropping parents in the Mississippi Delta emerged as a leader of civil rights activity in the early 1960s with her rallying message that she and all black people were "sick and tired of being sick and tired."[46]

Today the United States again faces a national health crisis, which has had a devastating impact on many communities, especially black communities in inner cities and rural districts. Current calls for the transformation of the health care system are not new; they are deeply rooted in the history of African-American health reform, which demonstrated the necessity of universal health provisions.

Part I

The Creation of a
Black Health Movement

1. Private Crusades for Public Health
Black Club Women and Public Health Work

Unwilling to accept the state of ill-health in black America at the turn of the twentieth century, black club women rallied around the cause of improving black health. Black women's community work for public health was consistent with the organized social welfare activities of women across the United States. Scholars have long noted black and white women's contributions to the creation of such institutions as churches, schools, hospitals, and public welfare agencies.[1] As the history of black club women shows, women's private efforts laid the community roots of public health work.

Black women built the infrastructure of their communities through their religious and secular associations, including church women's groups, female auxiliaries, and women's clubs. Club work was midway between the work of personal charity and professional social work and, as such, influenced the direction of social welfare work during the Progressive Era. Black club women, who numbered fewer than 5,000 in 1899 and over 300,000 in 1925, were at the center of social welfare work for African Americans. They acted on a wide range of issues, including education, housing, child care, and health. Black club women established day nurseries (all-day child care) and kindergartens in response to the needs of mothers in the labor force. They opened working girls' homes in the North and Midwest to assist young black southern migrants with housing, employment information, job training, and moral instruction.[2]

Much of their effort, however, focused on public health work because the very survival of African Americans was at stake. Segregation and racism resulted in the denial of basic health services to African Americans. High morbidity and mortality rates in black communities led black women to integrate health education and health care into the activities of local chapters of such organizations as the National Association of Colored Women, a national organization founded in 1896 to represent black club women. Public health work was important in black communities because racism led to a shortage of health professionals and medical institutions willing to serve African Americans. Even though curative medicine and technological advances have taken much of the credit for the increased longevity of human populations, preventive medicine and public health may have been more important, especially for black America.[3]

Private Crusades for Public Health

Black club women believed that health work was distinctively women's work because of their unquestioned acceptance of the gendered division of labor in the family, their commitment to racial uplift and alleviating poverty, and their concerns about sexual morality. As one club woman in Mississippi noted, club women were active in the public health field because "the responsibility for the health of the family is largely upon the women."[4]

Middle-class black women asserted that their class, as well as their gender, made them uniquely fitted to bring about the salvation of the race.[5] Acting on the assumption that good health was one characteristic of middle-class respectability, black club women set out to "clean up" the lives of the poor, imposing their own standards of appropriate behavior in their efforts for racial advancement.

Much of the history of black "self-help" has been that of the efforts of the black middle class to help the poor, motivated by self-interest as well as a sense of responsibility. Black middle-class women felt a personal stake in the "improvement" of the poor because of the potential effects on their own status. At issue for the middle class was the fact that white America did not recognize class differences among African Americans. "The status of the race is fixed by the impoverished conditions of the majority and not by the noble achievements of the ever increasing few," observed club woman Fannie Barrier Williams in 1904.[6] Mary Church Terrell, a member of the black elite who served as the first president of the National Association of Colored Women, warned club women to exercise caution in their actions toward the black poor:

> Colored women of education and culture know that they cannot escape altogether the consequences of the acts of their most depraved sisters. They see that even if they were wicked enough to turn a deaf ear to the call of duty, both policy and self-preservation demand that they go down among the lowly, the illiterate and even the vicious, to whom they are bound by the ties of race and sex, and put forth every possible effort to reclaim them.[7]

Black club women repeatedly expressed the sentiment that the fate of the middle class was tied to that of the poor, even as they sought to distinguish themselves from the black masses. The bonds of race that united black women did not erase class divisions. As historian Deborah White has argued, "black female unity was a political concept . . . not a social reality."[8]

Black middle-class women shared a vision of moral purity as an appropriate solution to racial advancement. Club women tried to spread their moral influence among poor women, emphasizing sexual restraint, in an effort to protect all black women from sexual danger. As the guardians of morality, club women insisted that black progress would only come about through their example. Their assertions of sexual respectability were black middle-class women's responses to racist sexual stereotypes. The notion that black women were by nature sexually promiscuous had long served as justification for white male access to black female bodies. To many white Americans, the rape of black women and the lynching of black men was simply no crime at all because of "the race's moral depravity." One of the major goals of the National Association of Colored Women was to address black women's sexual vulnerability by countering with positive, "moral" images of black women's sexuality.[9]

Club leaders repeatedly pointed to the historical origins of black woman's plight. "Slavery made her the only woman in America for whom virtue was not an ornament and a necessity," noted Williams.[10] Concern about sexual danger was common to many late nineteenth-century white women who challenged male sexual privilege. However, club women felt compelled to expose the sexual myths about black women while simultaneously decrying their real sexual abuse during and after slavery. Such complex motivations nevertheless cast sexually conservative overtones on otherwise progressive reform efforts in black communities.[11]

What follows, then, are illustrations of the organizational activities of middle-class black women within three major areas: the rural South, the urban South, and the urban North. The South was the heart of black America in the first half of the twentieth century. In 1910, of approximately ten million African Americans, 90 percent resided in the South. Most black health work was carried out by African Americans either in or from the South. Club women were especially active in the urban centers of the North and South where the organizational life of the black middle class was strongest and the migration of rural Southerners had steadily increased the black population and created pressing needs. On average, 6,700 black Southerners left the South annually from 1870 to 1890, and 15,000 annually from 1890 to 1910, with an exodus of about two million African Americans between 1890 and 1930. The result was that black health conditions became a nationwide concern.[12]

Black women's health projects in each of these three regions varied in scale, depending on available financial resources, but all attempted to compensate for the effects of poverty and institutionalized racism on black communities. In Chicago, community women's contributions to the establishment of Provident Hospital and Nurses' Training School demonstrate the key role of layworkers in creating and sustaining health institutions. In rural Alabama, the activities of the Tuskegee Woman's Club illustrate the influence of middle-class morals and manners on black women's attempts to uplift the poor and spread the "gospel of cleanliness." Finally, the projects of the Neighborhood Union in Atlanta indicate the importance of the community network through which club women collectively struggled for black health reform.

Provident Hospital and Nurses' Training School in Chicago

The urban North and Midwest held out the promise of escape from some of the worse aspects of southern life, including sharecropping, lynching, and rape. Chicago was one of the most popular destinations of migrating black Southerners. In 1890 it was the second largest American city, with over one million people.[13] Chicago was also home to Provident Hospital and Nurses' Training School, one of the 200 hospitals and nurse training schools established by African Americans across the country at the turn of the twentieth century. In this period, ethnic and religious groups commonly organized their own hospitals to meet the needs of their communities.[14]

Black club women, a few of whom were doctors, created health institutions in their communities. Although historians have provided insightful analysis of the development of black hospitals and nursing schools, they have focused primarily on the role of black health professionals, especially doctors and nurses.[15] Scholars have paid insufficient attention to the contributions of laywomen to the founding and maintenance of hospitals and nursing schools.

The early history of Provident Hospital and Nurses' Training School in Chicago, one of the best-studied black hospitals, demonstrates the importance of the uncompensated labor of laywomen who helped to sustain such institutions across the country. Laywomen's approach was characterized by a sweeping vision of health care that informed their belief that the cook's knife was as important to the running of the hospital as the surgeon's knife and that nurses were as important to the recovery of patients as physicians.[16]

Provident Hospital, which opened in 1891 with twelve beds in a three-story house, was the first black-controlled hospital in the United States and a major institution in Chicago's black community.[17] Dr. Daniel Hale Williams, a black doctor who performed one of the first successful open-heart surgeries, was the founder of Provident Hospital.[18] As early as 1888 he had envisioned opening a hospital that would not discriminate against African Americans, but plans did not get underway until Emma Reynolds arrived in Chicago in 1890. Reynolds, a young black woman from Kansas City, hoped to enroll in a nurses' training school in Chicago, but all the schools rejected her because she was an African American.[19] A number of people attempted to get her accepted, including her brother the Reverend Louis H. Reynolds and Daniel Williams, but to no avail. Williams decided that if the "color line" could not be broken, the only solution was to open a nursing school for black women with an adjoining hospital.

People had a variety of motives for establishing Provident Hospital and Nurses' Training School. Black residents of Chicago supported the hospital because it provided much needed health care to some 15,000 African Americans who were denied treatment at local white hospitals, with the exception of Cook County Hospital.[20] Black doctors, such as Williams, supported Provident Hospital in order to assist black people and at the same time meet the physicians' own professional needs. Denied admitting privileges at white hospitals, African-American physicians needed the hospital as a place to bring their patients and gain clinical experience.[21]

Middle-class black women, such as Fannie Barrier Williams, supported Provident in order to assist poor women and children and to advance the position of black womanhood. Fannie Williams (no relation to Daniel Williams), may have learned about the proposed hospital and nursing school from her pastor at the All Souls Unitarian Church, from whom Daniel Williams had solicited assistance.[22] Fannie Williams (1855–1944), who moved to Chicago in 1887 from New York after marrying lawyer S. Laing Williams, was a prominent national club leader and journalist. She had been a teacher to freedpeople in the South after the Civil War and later taught in the schools in Washington, D.C. In Chicago she served on the board of a number of civic institutions, including the Frederick Douglass Center settlement project, the Phyllis Wheatley Home for working women and girls, and the Illinois Woman's Alliance, and as the first African American and first woman on the Chicago Library Board.[23]

Even though Daniel Williams touted Provident Hospital as a project of interracial cooperation with no color barrier, Fannie Williams was adamant that the nursing school be reserved only for black women because of the racial restrictions elsewhere. Provident's nursing school was only the second in the country for black women, with the first having been established at Spelman College in Atlanta in 1886.[24] By 1914 the Provident nursing school graduated 118 women from twenty-four states, including Emma Reynolds (class of 1892), who went on to earn an M.D. in Texas and open a medical practice in New Orleans.[25]

Community women hoped that the nursing school would expand employment opportunities for black women, given the high percentage of them in the paid workforce. There were very few job options, aside from teaching, for black women seeking professional careers at the turn of the century. Nursing provided young women with an attractive alternative to domestic service work, often the mainstay of black female employment. For example, by 1910 over 75 percent of all black women workers in Chicago were employed in domestic work. Even though nursing still had negative associations with service work, many black women believed that nursing would provide better paid and more respected work for black women. The nursing school met the goals of young black women seeking better jobs, the requirements of the hospital for inexpensive staffing, and the desire of middle-class black women to "uplift" young women and elevate black womanhood.[26]

While Daniel Williams led the efforts to establish Provident, black women presided over most of the community organizing and fund-raising work, tasks that were essential to the survival of all voluntary institutions. Fannie Williams became "official solicitor" for the hospital and continued in this role until 1896. Early organizing meetings were held at the home of Chicago leader Mrs. J. C. Plummer, later Vice President of the Chicago Anti-Lynching Committee. The attending women formed two "ladies' auxiliaries," one for the west and one for the south side of the city. One particularly popular fund-raiser, an evening of entertainment directed by Mrs. Cora Scott Pond Pope, collected $1,300.[27]

Some of black women's political energy went into raising money from wealthy white Chicagoans, a few of whom did donate thousands of dollars to Provident. For example, nurse Nanahyoke Sockum Curtis, married to Provident Hospital's first intern, was influential in convincing meatpacking giant Philip D. Armour to contribute to Provident. Other wealthy whites who gave money included George M. Pullman of the railcar industry and department store merchant Marshall Field. These businessmen stood to benefit from the hospital because some of the patients treated there came as a result of accidents incurred at the railways and stockyards owned by these men.[28]

Most of the donors, however, were African Americans, among the poorest people in the city. One cannot overestimate the sacrifice of those who donated and collected these dollars. Even though prominent national leaders such as Frederick Douglass, Booker T. Washington, W. E. B. Du Bois, and Ida B. Wells-Barnett publicly endorsed Provident Hospital, it was the local community that sustained it. As one national black club leader pointed out, black women's voluntary contributions were indeed noteworthy "when one reflects that few Negro women are women of leisure, or, of large means; and that the time and money they give to public work is usually at a sacrifice practically unknown to the women of other races engaged in similar work."[29] Even though white contributions were vital in the early years, black people "provided an ever larger portion of Provident's operational expenses and 90 per cent of its endowment."[30]

Laywomen, as both individuals and representatives of their churches and clubs, donated the majority of basic goods and services to Provident Hospital and Nurses' Training School. Churches were especially important as the center of black community life and the springboard for the development of secular women's clubs. Black churches, with their predominantly female members, held fund-raisers and furnished the hospital with cots.[31] Women made small cash donations and contributed everything from fruit, coffee, bread, and ice cream to a parlor stove and a clothes wringer. Community women formed linen clubs to make the institution more comfortable and home-like. They provided lace for nurses' caps and furnishings for nurses' rooms, and they made sheets, pillowcases, towels, and tablecloths for the hospital and nursing school. The value of such items did not go unnoticed by the trustees of Provident, who saw fit to publish long, detailed lists of donors' names and their contributions in the annual reports of the hospital, no doubt to encourage their continued support. For example, Provident's first annual report in 1892 provided a monthly accounting several pages long detailing the donations, over 90 percent from women.[32]

The accumulation of each small contribution saved Provident money over the years. In addition, such gifts no doubt encouraged favorable impressions of the hospital among patients, nurses, and doctors. Good publicity was essential to an institution struggling to establish its own legitimacy, especially at a time when many people still associated hospitals with almshouses and places one went to die.

Community women's maintenance of the infrastructure of Provident became even greater when they institutionalized their role in the administration of the hospital by forming the official Woman's Auxiliary Board in 1896.[33] Women may have created their own separate organization after being squeezed out of their previous role on the regular advisory board, where at least four women had served, including journalist, club woman, and antilynching crusader Ida B. Wells-Barnett. The Woman's Auxiliary Board, with the wives of hospital staff among its membership, spent most of its time on fund-raising. The efforts of seventy board members resulted in thousands of dollars' worth of goods, everything from surgical tools and equipment to a vacuum sweeper and kitchen utensils. For laywomen, no item was outside the boundary of hospital and nursing school maintenance if it kept Provident running smoothly. In 1911, no doubt to encourage the continuation of such voluntary work, the trustees admitted that "were it not for the efforts of this band of noble women . . . it would indeed be difficult to surmise the fate of the institution itself."[34]

The female board members expanded their efforts beyond the walls of the hospital into public health programs designed to lower high infant mortality rates and improve the health of children. Concern for children, a major theme of Progressive Era reformers, led to the development of a national child welfare movement.[35] Female reformers believed that bettering the lives of children would ensure healthier, more productive adults, and middle-class women were drawn to helping the children of the poor. Black women, in particular, argued that the survival and uplift of the race depended on healthy children.[36]

The Woman's Auxiliary Board tried to expand children's access to good nutrition and a clean environment through pure milk and fresh air, typical health programs in the urban North. In 1910 the Woman's Auxiliary Board took over leadership of Provident's infant feeding program in order to provide free pure milk to babies in poor black neighborhoods.[37] Milk programs — a popular public health strategy for addressing high infant mortality rates — were especially needed for black infants, whose mortality rate was generally twice that of white infants. Indeed, several milk programs began in Chicago after a 1903 commission found problems with the production and distribution of the city's milk.[38]

In 1911 the Woman's Auxiliary Board initiated a second public health program for children when it erected a "fresh air tent" on the roof of Provident Hospital. A number of voluntary groups in Chicago set up children's tents or "fresh air stations" in poor neighborhoods so that sick children, especially those with tuberculosis, could receive nursing care outside crowded tenement houses. Erected during the summertime, the tent provided a place where "scores of babies find in hot weather their only chance for life."[39]

Throughout Provident's early history it is evident that black hospitals depended on the unpaid labor of laywomen. Women linked Provident to the black communities of Chicago through their auxiliaries and clubs. Through endless organizing and fund-raising, community women tried to sustain a service they saw as vital to the health needs of African Americans. Furthermore, Provident became the focus of much of the charity work of the black community, work primarily carried out by the organizational activities of middle-class black women.[40]

Tuskegee Woman's Club of Alabama

Government public health officials generally ignored African Americans in the rural South, so black club women and other black reformers integrated public health work into their rural development projects. Members of the Tuskegee Woman's Club, associated with Tuskegee Institute in Macon County, Alabama, provided health education as part of their social welfare work among the agricultural workers on plantations in the surrounding countryside. Many African Americans in the rural South were sharecroppers working on white-owned plantations where the entire family was involved in the production of a cash crop, such as cotton. Sanitation was difficult at best, with open wells and outdoor privies (toilets), and malnutrition was a serious problem. In response, the Tuskegee Woman's Club established a social settlement, which was similar to the settlement houses created in the North to aid immigrants. Middle-class ideals shaped the club's educational mission among the rural poor.[41]

Black women's clubs were typically dominated by educators. Members of the Tuskegee Woman's Club, such as Margaret Murray Washington, were teachers or the wives of teachers at Tuskegee Institute. Margaret Washington (1865–1925), head of the Tuskegee Woman's Club from 1895 to 1925, was a teacher and the third wife of Booker T. Washington, who led Tuskegee Institute. Under her guidance club membership grew from 13 to

130 by 1920.[42] Margaret Washington was born in Mississippi and graduated from Fisk University, a black liberal arts college in Tennessee. In the early 1890s she joined Tuskegee Institute as Lady Principal in charge of female students and married Booker T. Washington. She was a club leader at the national and state level, and she became president of the National Association of Colored Women in 1898 and president of the Alabama State Federation of Colored Women's Clubs in 1900.[43]

Black educational institutions, such as Tuskegee Institute, Hampton Institute, and Fisk University, provided the support and stimulus for much of black women's social service activity. These schools reinforced an urgent sense of duty to others and an obligation to assist the poor.[44] Janie Porter Barrett, who served as president of the Virginia State Federation of Colored Women's Clubs and founded a social settlement, reported that during her time attending Hampton Institute in Virginia she felt burdened by an overwhelming sense of responsibility to her race. As students, Barrett recalled, "we were always hearing about our duty to our race, and I got so tired of that! Why, on Sundays I used to wake up and say to myself, 'To-day I don't have to do a single thing for my race!' "[45]

At Tuskegee Institute students learned it was their duty to the race to uphold moral purity and maintain cleanliness. Both Margaret Washington and Booker T. Washington supported a racial uplift agenda that called for people to be clean in mind, body, and soul. The Tuskegee philosophy equated sexual respectability with moral cleanliness. For example, Tuskegee sociologist Monroe Nathan Work criticized the absence of restraint in the behavior of local people before the arrival of Tuskegee's influence. Work complained that people had participated in a popular annual camp-meeting held near Tuskegee Institute, and that

> there was much about this meeting that was demoralizing and immoral. Whiskey in large quantities was sold in the near by woods. There was a loosening of moral restraints and the people were generally debauched.[46]

Meanwhile, the Tuskegee philosophy opposed sexual and alcoholic indulgence.

At the Annual Tuskegee Negro Conference, which began in 1892, black educators tried to alter the behavior of the rural poor. Washington claimed that the conferences were simply a forum for rural black people to discuss their problems and identify solutions, but he pushed his own vision of how to solve rural black poverty. He wanted to create independent, self-sufficient farmers who raised their own food on their own land, lived in nice homes, were free from debt, and led "respectable" lives.[47]

Hundreds, eventually thousands, of rural African Americans attended the Annual Tuskegee Negro Conference, which drew regional attention. After a few years, Tuskegee added a "Workers' Day" to the one-day farmers' conference as an opportunity for teachers, ministers, nurses, social workers, and extension service agents to discuss solutions to the problems of rural African Americans. Early in the twentieth century the Annual Tuskegee Negro Conference included a health component, with lectures by state and federal public health officials, health exhibits, and free physical examinations by nurses.[48]

The annual conferences stressed the significance of women's influence on the physical and moral health of their families. In targeting women, participants even suggested that women should set a proper example for their families and dress and behave modestly in public. It was up to rural women, they argued, to insist on living in cabins with more than one room, presumably because children should not witness their parents' sexual activity. They urged women to help lower black mortality rates by providing proper clothing, food, and a clean home for their families, implying that women's irresponsibility, not financial constraints, had jeopardized the lives of their children.[49]

Such attitudes informed much of the activities of the Tuskegee Woman's Club, especially in its work with the poor on plantations and in small towns surrounding the school. In fact the club was established by Margaret Washington, who resented the fact that her husband did not permit women to speak at the annual conferences. In 1897 the club established the Elizabeth Russell Settlement on the nearby Russell Plantation, where the people were "among the most backward in the county."[50] The club women tried to improve the physical, spiritual, moral, and educational life of the hundreds of residents. Many of the people had been released from jails in Macon County to work out their time in agricultural labor on the plantation, a common exploitative southern practice known as the convict lease system. At the plantation, people lived in small cabins that had survived from the days of slavery. They "had little or no idea of the proper way in which to bring up their children," explained Margaret Washington, and "they had little or no idea of the sort of food necessary for the body; they gave little or no thought to their moral or spiritual life." Legal marriage did not concern them, and they "had simply been left to themselves to drift, without training, guidance, or help from the plantation owners."[51] In the eyes of the club women, it was a population in desperate need of help.

The club women's solution was education. They sent Tuskegee graduate Ann Davis to open a school for the children on the plantation. For twelve years club women taught at the plantation every weekend until residents could run the programs themselves. They organized a Sunday school, boys' clubs, girls' sewing classes, mothers' clubs, and newspaper reading clubs for men. In 1920 Margaret Washington boasted that as a result of the work of the club women, the people on the plantation had become "a pride to themselves and a pride to those of us who have given our time."[52] Even more effusive in praise, Mary Church Terrell indicated that the club women had performed "the work of bringing the light of knowledge and the gospel of cleanliness to their poor benighted sisters on the plantations."[53]

Like black women's clubs elsewhere, the Tuskegee Woman's Club focused on the home as an important site for reform work. As black club woman Sarah Dudley Pettey explained, "Home life is the citadel and bulwark of every race's moral life."[54] The club sent members into homes in the town of Tuskegee to promote cleanliness, personal hygiene, thrift, proper manners and morals, and good homemaking and mothering skills. In 1911 Dr. John Kenney, medical director of the hospital at Tuskegee, described this house-to-house uplift activity by members of the Tuskegee Woman's Club:

> The smallest details are looked after, as how to prepare and serve their food, how and when to bathe, how to ventilate their houses, how to care for their hair, the washing of their clothing, cleaning of their teeth, sleeping between sheets, and all such subjects as tend to improve their home conditions. The special subjects of tuberculosis and typhoid fever have been discussed before the people in the most elementary manner possible.[55]

The women even paid for dental care for a hundred children and purchased new toothbrushes. Health and welfare work, with all its middle-class trappings, was a hallmark of the reform activity of black club women.

Cleanliness and improved health were not antagonistic to the interests of the poor, who no doubt had their own reasons to support health reform. However, some may have objected to the invasive manner in which their lives were scrutinized. Tuskegee residents apparently made a point to carefully clean up the inside and outside of their homes before a visit from Margaret Washington and the other club women.[56] Club women's records indicate that the women presumed that the recipients welcomed and benefited from their reform activity, but such sources are less forthcoming about the meanings of such work for those they aided. Poor black women no doubt benefited from public health work because it relieved them of some of the labor of keeping their families alive, but it also increased their burden by insisting that it was women's responsibility to meet the appropriate standards of cleanliness and respectability.

Neighborhood Union of Atlanta

The health work of the Neighborhood Union of Atlanta, an organization established in 1908 under the leadership of Lugenia Burns Hope, illustrates how club women drew on community networks to convey their messages about cleanliness and their critiques of inequality in the urban South.[57] Through the Union, which provided the first public health programs for African Americans in Atlanta, faculty wives of Spelman and Morehouse colleges along with other local women organized lectures on cleanliness and health care, investigated the sanitary conditions of homes and streets in black neighborhoods, and enacted what historian Jacqueline Rouse called "the moral cleanup of the community."[58]

Lugenia Burns Hope (1871–1947) was the central force behind the establishment of the Neighborhood Union, which she led for twenty-five years. Hope grew up in St. Louis, Missouri, and Chicago, where she worked with the famous Hull House settlement. In 1897 she married John Hope and a year later moved to Atlanta, where he eventually became president of Morehouse College. Inspired by W. E. B. Du Bois and the Atlanta University conferences, Hope committed herself to social welfare work for women and children. She took part in most of the major social reform, black feminist, and racial uplift organizations of her day. She was linked to the national network of black female leaders that included Fannie Barrier Williams and Margaret Murray Washington.

By the first decade of the twentieth century Atlanta was a segregated city, where the black population was excluded from certain parks, hotels, and restaurants. Most black Atlantans, 40 percent of the city's population, lived in small wooden shacks built on piles of bricks in alley communities. Much like in other southern cities, African-American living quarters were in these poorly drained hollows behind white houses where city filth accumulated. Black neighborhoods in the urban South were low priorities for local government development of such amenities as sewers, adequate water, and paved streets. Not surprisingly, such living conditions contributed to the fact that black mortality rates were 70 percent higher than white, especially for tuberculosis and infant mortality.[59]

It is in this context that the club women of the Neighborhood Union began their public health work. They created the Neighborhood Union health center, which was part of a nationwide neighborhood health center movement that began in the United States about 1910 on the premise that health professionals could best reach people in their own communities.[60] The Union held its first health clinic in 1908, and by 1930 over 4,000 people relied on the basic health services it provided.[61] From 1917 to 1921 neighborhood volunteers assisted the Union with a housing survey that documented the absence of city services, including the lack of streetlights, as well as inadequate garbage removal, water supplies, and toilet facilities.

Much of the success of the Neighborhood Union was due to the women's direct contact with local people and their ongoing efforts to involve the community in the projects. Women organized the work of the Union into sixteen zones in the city, each of which had a chairwoman and ten female supervisors. Each of the supervisors appointed ten other women to assist them, therefore providing every zone with 110 women workers, for a total of over 1,700 women volunteers. Also, students from local black colleges increased the number of assistants as they aided the health campaigns through inspecting homes for sanitary conditions. In 1919 some 140 volunteers inspected 5,400 homes. The neighborhood campaigns and projects in schools resulted in contacts with some 45,000 people, approximately three-fourths of the black population in Atlanta.[62]

The women of the Neighborhood Union used their elaborate organizational structure to facilitate the participation of much of Atlanta's black population in National Negro Health Week activities. Across the nation, club women successfully mobilized community support for National Negro Health Week, an annual black health celebration that began in 1915 (see Chapter 2). Dr. Mary Fitzbutler Waring, a physician and school teacher in Chicago, urged laywomen to get involved in public health work even if they had no medical expertise. In her capacity as head of the health and hygiene department of the National Association of Colored Women, Waring encouraged club women to create black health campaigns in their neighborhoods. Waring, who earned two medical degrees and was elected president of the association in 1933, wrote frequent articles on public health for the black club women's journal *National Notes*. In 1917 she urged club women to organize observances of National Negro Health Week to help the poor, and to "go into the backways and the tenement houses, into the alleys and basements, into the places unfrequented by garbage wagons and street cleaners and here help teach and preach 'cleanliness.'" She explained that "the work of cleaning up does not require a learned discourse on streptococcipyogenses aurem or any other microbe, — it just means soap, water, screens and energy."[63]

The Neighborhood Union did not operate National Negro Health Week observances alone; it persuaded a wide range of black and white organizations to join together to improve the health of the city.[64] The Union oversaw the actual implementation of the plans under the black health week slogan, "Burn, Bury and Beautify." For each observance of Negro Health Week beginning in 1915, the women of the Union provided health lectures at schools and churches, films, and distributed thousands of health pamphlets, often door to door. They targeted the unsanitary conditions of businesses owned by white merchants in black neighborhoods, and they directed the clean-up work of boys and girls, who turned unsafe vacant lots into playgrounds. They also created medical and dental clinics, including a clinic in 1917 that traveled for sixteen weeks around the city providing health services to poor black people.[65]

In 1929 Atlanta held its most elaborate National Negro Health Week observance, under the auspices of the Neighborhood Union with wide support from the community, including schools, churches, black women's clubs, the city health department, insurance agencies, and numerous voluntary organizations. Many people helped to organize the event, including the twenty-one members of the executive committee. Over 200 employees heard health lectures at four industrial plants, 9,000 people heard lectures at churches, and 10,500 children heard lectures at schools, where organizers selected a boy and girl as "Mr. and Miss Health." According to Atlanta's health week report,

> A monster parade through downtown streets climaxed the health week observance participated in by fully 1,000 boys and girls, public school pupils bearing banners and posters with appropriate slogans for the promotion of better health.[66]

Forrester B. Washington, director of the Atlanta University School of Social Work, wrote in praise of the campaign:

> I know the claims of a lot of other cities and I know how much of their programs are simply on paper, but if you could have seen these activities in Atlanta as I saw them first-hand, I believe you would feel as I do — that this was the most complete Negro Health Week achievement so far.[67]

The type of grassroots support illustrated by Atlanta's black health campaigns was only possible because of middle-class women's efforts to involve poor black people in this neighborhood work.

The community health activism of the Neighborhood Union preceded the development of government-led health programs for African Americans in Atlanta. The women of the Union used their volunteer health work to try to stimulate government interest in the plight of black Americans; they exerted political pressure on the city government by petitioning it to extend city services to segregated black neighborhoods. The Union succeeded in obtaining municipal action to secure improvements on twenty streets, including repairs in lighting and plumbing. In 1929 the Negro Health Week executive committee even presented the Atlanta city council with suggestions on ways to improve housing conditions and health facilities in the form of a proposed amendment to the city building codes and a rooming house law.[68] Through organizations like the Neighborhood Union, laywomen kept some of the basic survival issues of black people before government officials.

Conclusion

Black women were at the forefront of community health work for African Americans at the turn of the twentieth century, a time when layworkers led black public health activities.[69] Black women turned to their clubs and auxiliaries to provide public health services that would have been otherwise unavailable. Women's voluntary work for Provident Hospital and Nurses' Training School in Chicago, the Tuskegee Woman's Club in Alabama, and the Neighborhood Union in Atlanta was typical of the organizational activity of black women campaigning for public welfare. Despite staff and budget limitations, they provided health education and some basic health services that enriched impoverished communities. In Chicago and Atlanta, women reformers tried to provide to African Americans the urban amenities that white people often received from tax-supported city services. In rural communities like Tuskegee, women used educational programs for both black children and adults as their primary tool for self-development and racial advancement. In each case, black club women demonstrated a willingness to perform the tedious, day-to-day tasks involved in fundraising and health promotion. Taken together, the local activities of organized black women laid the groundwork for the black health movement.

2. Spreading the Gospel of Health
Tuskegee Institute and National Negro Health Week

In the early twentieth century the health reform efforts of black club women became part of a national black health movement. In 1915 Booker T. Washington, the most powerful black leader of his time, launched a health education campaign known as National Negro Health Week from Tuskegee Institute in Alabama. Washington, as founder and head of the school, had long emphasized sanitation and hygiene in his educational work. However, that year he set in motion a health campaign that would grow into a nationwide black health movement over the next thirty-five years. For black leaders and community organizers, National Negro Health Week campaigns provided a way to advance the race through the promotion of black health education and cooperation across racial lines.

Faith in the power of education and the possibilities for intergroup cooperation were typical of early twentieth-century beliefs about social change and were hallmarks of progressivism. Indeed, the emphasis on public education and cooperation between voluntary organizations and health departments marked the emergence of the "new public health" after 1910.[1] The emphasis on education and interracial cooperation was also characteristic of black activism in the early twentieth century, as seen in the work of black club women, and the early development of the National Urban League, a black social service organization.[2]

National Negro Health Week was a far-reaching but little-known feature of the educational work of Tuskegee Institute, which was "the center of things relating to the Negro."[3] Tuskegee's leaders promoted National Negro Health Week activity among black and white organizations and brought black health problems to the attention of the federal government. Meanwhile, community members, health workers, and educators, especially graduates of Tuskegee Institute, developed local observances and spread the movement across the South and the nation. Tuskegee Institute served as headquarters for National Negro Health Week from 1915 to 1930, at which point the United States Public Health Service (USPHS) took over the campaign and turned it into a year-round program.

On the national level, black men were the prominent leaders of the National Negro Health Week movement, while on the local level, black women continued their previous health reform tradition and carried out much of the community organizing. The movement nationalized black health activities that had existed since at least the late nineteenth century, especially in the public welfare work of black women. Under Tuskegee's leadership, black men were drawn into black health campaigns through their professional and business organizations. Women had more opportunity to exert their influence at the local level, where they did the less glamorous grassroots work behind the scenes and within local health week planning committees.

Black health activists turned National Negro Health Week into a vehicle for social welfare organizing and political activity in a period when the vast majority of African Americans were without formal political and economic power. Much like white social reformers of the early twentieth century, black reformers turned to government and charity organizations to ensure the permanency of their volunteer efforts. Unlike their white counterparts, however, black activists found only limited government and private resources available for health promotion in their communities.

The history of the movement illustrates how at least some African Americans pursued improved health by making political claims on the state. Their activity politicized black health needs and therefore indirectly advocated social rights. The emphasis on "needs" rather than "rights" was a politically conscious choice in the era of Jim Crow, when Booker T. Washington and many African Americans doubted the efficacy of rights rhetoric for social change. Nevertheless, in this context the assertion of black health needs was itself political expression. The danger of a "needs" discourse approach was that, historically, white Americans had not perceived black needs as a political priority and indeed had legislated against them.[4]

Because black Americans received a vastly unequal share in the segregated system, black activists tried to shape the direction of the growing welfare state to ensure that it addressed black interests. The historical denial of black humanity and the white belief that African Americans were a degenerating people, if not headed for outright extinction, meant that it was crucial for African Americans to retain control over the right to define their needs.[5] African Americans waged similar struggles for inclusion and autonomy in the first half of the twentieth century through other social movements, including the black education movement, black hospital movement, and black birth control movement.[6] Summing up the goals of the black health movement, Eugene Kinckle Jones of the National Urban League concluded that "the Negro's struggle for health might be considered an effort of the race to survive."[7]

The Tuskegee Connection: Booker T. Washington and the Creation of National Negro Health Week

Booker T. Washington (1856–1915) had a knack for building on the work of others by expanding on their visions through his access to the political and economic power of white elites and a large following of black supporters. Born a slave on a small Virginia farm, Washington went on to graduate from Hampton Institute in Virginia, a school that provided teacher training and industrial education through a philosophy of Christianity, thrift, and hard work. In 1881 Washington founded Tuskegee Institute, modeled on Hampton, which became one of the most famous black institutions in America. Even critics of Washington, such as the black Harvard graduate W. E. B. Du Bois, acknowledged the formidable power and influence of the "Tuskegee Machine" that Washington had built up through his connections to northern philanthropists, white politicians, and members of the black middle class.[8]

Historians have classified early twentieth-century black political strategy as following one of two opposing approaches: the Booker T. Washington accommodation model, which emphasized economic self-help, and the W. E. B. Du Bois integration model, best exemplified by the National Association for the Advancement of Colored People (NAACP), which argued for the primacy of black civil rights.[9] Although these men came to symbolize different approaches to the struggle against racism, black activists and social movements rarely operated exclusively within one or the other framework.

Indeed, Washington and Du Bois differed from each other much less than their popularized images would suggest. Historians and contemporaries criticized Washington for appearing to surrender to southern racism and promoting black subordination by asking black people to accept a place at the bottom of the southern racial hierarchy and economy. Meanwhile, Du Bois seemed to ignore the immediate survival needs of the black rural poor in his emphasis on voting rights and the development of a college educated "talented tenth."[10] Yet, both Washington and Du Bois sought to train a cadre of black leaders, and both saw improved health and educational opportunities as part of the foundation for black emancipation. Despite the association of Negro Health Week with the work of Washington, individual members of the NAACP actively supported it. Du Bois himself was even a keynote speaker for at least one black health week program.[11]

PRECURSORS TO A NATIONAL BLACK HEALTH WEEK CAMPAIGN

Washington developed the idea for a black health observance from a successful black health program created by the Negro Organization Society of Virginia. Members of the Negro Organization Society, many of whom were Hampton Institute graduates, believed that health promotion was one of the cornerstones upon which an uplifted race depended. Their motto for improving the status of African Americans was to develop better farms, homes, education, and health.

The Negro Organization Society was founded about 1910 to unite groups interested in black advancement. The society was a coalition of over 250 black religious and secular organizations, representing 350,000 African Americans in Virginia, about half of the state's black population. In 1912 the society launched a clean-up day throughout the state, recruiting support from the Virginia Board of Health, and in 1913 and 1914 it expanded the health campaign into a health week project.[12]

Robert Russa Moton (1867–1940), who worked at Hampton Institute for several years, was president of the society. Moton, son of a slave, graduated from Hampton Institute in 1890. After returning to visit his home in rural Virginia from Hampton, Moton recalled: "I was convinced that whatever else I might do, there was nothing more worth while than helping just such people in just that kind of a community."[13] He was active in the National Urban League and the National Negro Business League, a black business organization established in 1900 by Washington to promote economic self-sufficiency. After Washington's death, Moton became his successor at Tuskegee Institute.

Washington also drew on the political experience and public health activity of sociologist Monroe Nathan Work (1866–1945). Work earned a master's degree in 1903 from the University of Chicago. In 1905, while teaching at a college in Savannah, Georgia, he helped develop a citywide health campaign for African Americans in which a black men's club in Savannah carried "the gospel of health" to the community. During his years in Georgia, Work joined with Du Bois in the civil rights work of the Niagara Movement, precursor to the NAACP. Work also assisted Du Bois on the 1906 publication *The Health Physique of the Negro American*.[14] In 1908

Washington hired Work to head the new Department of Records and Research at Tuskegee Institute in order to study the historical and contemporary conditions of black people in America and to provide Washington with accurate data for his speeches and writings.

The topic of health was a major focus of Work's research. Work relied on statistics, long a favored method of public health reformers and sociologists, to gather quantitative, "objective" evidence about the poor state of black health conditions.[15] He was an empiricist who believed in the power of cold hard facts to influence opinion because, as he once said, "you can't argue with facts." The key to social change, he determined, was "to get the facts about the Negro before the country."[16]

Work believed that public forums were essential in the effort to improve black health conditions. By 1909 he succeeded in having health sessions at the Annual Tuskegee Negro Conference, a forum for local black farmers, educators, and social welfare workers to discuss social problems affecting rural African Americans. Thousands of people attended these conferences. Most importantly, in the 1914 conference Work presented a series of charts that contained disturbing statistics on black health conditions in the South.[17] "Mr. Work had some estimated figures that rather shocked the colored people of the country," recalled Tuskegee leader Albon Holsey.[18] Work's health statistics had an impact well beyond the conference and attracted national attention when black and white newspapers reported his findings.

Work's statistical compilations provided evidence to confirm what some health leaders had long believed, that African Americans had exceedingly high morbidity and mortality rates. Challenging those whites who argued that these high rates were a sign of inherent racial inferiority, Work argued that nearly half of all black deaths were premature and could have been prevented through public health efforts. He also pointed out the monetary as well as human costs of this tragedy, estimating that sickness and death among black people cost the South $300,000,000 annually. Thus, poor black health not only reduced the quality and length of life of African Americans but also resulted in an economic burden on the South as a whole. Earlier, white statistician Frederick L. Hoffman had argued that the racial degeneration of the black population was a serious hindrance to the economic progress of whites. Now, Work advanced the same argument but for an entirely different purpose: to promote the necessity of black health reform. "At the same time that our appalling health conditions were pointed out," explained Work, "attention was called to the possibility of health improvement," primarily through application of sanitary science and preventive medicine.[19]

Launching National Negro Health Week

By 1914 Washington was convinced that the time was right to launch a major black health campaign, given the public interest in Work's findings and the success of Virginia's black health program. Washington informed Moton that he had plans to start his own health campaign. "I do not want to interfere with your own plans," explained Washington, "but rather to emphasize what you have been doing so well in Virginia."[20] Since Moton offered no objection, Washington convinced Anson Phelps Stokes, a northern industrial philanthropist, to donate $500 from the Phelps-Stokes Fund toward publicity costs for the campaign.[21]

In Washington's 1915 "call" for a Negro Health Week observance, which he signed as head of the National Negro Business League, he asserted that racial advancement and economic prosperity required both good health and black unity:

> Without health . . . it will be impossible for us to have permanent success in business, in property getting, [and] in acquiring education. . . . Without health and long life all else fails.

Continuing, Washington avowed:

> We must reduce our high death-rate, dethrone disease and enthrone health and long life. We may differ on other subjects, but there is no room for difference here. Let us make a strong, long united pull together.[22]

He hoped for widespread support despite political differences among African Americans.

Washington's urgent message struck a responsive chord. His proposal received the endorsement of a wide range of national black organizations, including those representing black doctors, nurses, teachers, and club women. Work, who was responsible for promoting National Negro Health Week through the Department of Records and Research, contacted state health officers and state education directors, many of whom responded positively to the vigorous promotional effort. Black health week received favorable coverage in the white and black press, especially in southern cities.

Hundreds of letters and newsclippings poured into Tuskegee Institute, attesting to the presence of black health week programs across the country. In all, sixteen states held health week activities that first year, especially in the South. The community efforts to organize National Negro Health Week programs did unite individuals and organizations interested in the welfare of black people and brought a degree of cooperation across and within racial lines.[23]

Germ Theory and the Color Line: Politics, Segregation, and Health

Black leaders such as Washington and Moton used the promotion of black health to criticize segregation and advance black rights. Washington was no mere accommodationist, and, backed by Monroe Work's sociological data, he waged an ideological battle over the impact of segregation on health. Washington preached that segregation was hazardous to health and resulted in a no-win situation: it promoted sickness among black people and failed to protect the health of white people. In his closing address for Baltimore's Negro Health Week observance, he lectured to some 3,000 African Americans, along with a few white people, who had crowded into the Bethel A.M.E. Church.[24] In his speech, Washington critiqued the practice of segregation, stating that it was unnecessary and unjust, and left African Americans without adequate health provisions. As he explained elsewhere, it was wrong that black people did not have "proper streets, sewerage, lighting and other modern conveniences and necessities, . . . notwithstanding, in many cases, they pay a large proportion of the taxes that provide for the city government." He asserted that "before we go far in segregating the Negro we should study the effects of segregation upon the Indian," drawing an explicit parallel to the colonization of American Indians and the deadly consequences of the reservation system.[25]

Not all black leaders agreed on the extent to which segregation was the cause rather than the result of unhealthy black living conditions. Although black newspapers often published articles to demonstrate that segregation forced African Americans to live in the most unimproved and unsanitary parts of cities, a 1915 editorial in a black St. Louis newspaper blamed poor black people for segregation. In a morally chastising tone, the author stated that segregation would end only when black people cleaned up their homes. A respectable appearance, according to this argument, would counter white justifications for segregation and claims that black homes were run-down and that they depreciated white property values. "Poverty is no excuse for dirt or disease," concluded the editorial.[26]

Black leaders such as Washington challenged the rhetoric of segregation by unpacking its assumptions about racial isolation in the face of scientific understanding of germ theory. Washington and Moton asserted that black and white health problems, like black and white lives, were not separate but deeply interconnected. Black leaders used germ theory to their own political ends. They pointed out that because germs did not respect segregation, white people were at risk for contracting diseases from black people. Although black leaders were motivated by the belief that good health was a universal right, they argued that it was in the interests of white people to safeguard black health.

Booker T. Washington knew how to couch his politics in a language that white Americans would hear. To that end, he carried out a campaign to solicit white support for black health improvement by warning that "germs know no color line."[27] In effect, he applied social relations to germ theory and invoked the threat of cross-racial contagion. Germ theory, which grew out of the discoveries of bacteriology in the late nineteenth century, focused on identifying disease-causing agents. The idea that germs caused diseases became a part of the popular understanding of illness, leading to public concern that individual sick people could transmit diseases to others.

GERMS KNOW NO COLOR LINE:
DOMESTIC SERVANTS AND DISEASE TRANSMISSION

Black leaders, including Washington and Moton, preached the dangers of disease by emphasizing the hazards of an unhealthy black workforce to white employers. This approach was similar to Work's statistical presentation of the ramifications of black illness on the economy of the South. The South's need for black labor meant that white Southerners could not ignore the need to improve black health.

Ironically, in conveying the message that germs crossed the color line, Washington and Moton told stories that targeted black women as the primary culprits of disease transmission to whites. Storytelling was a well-known Washington trademark, used for the purposes of entertainment and education. Usually tales were about the follies of ignorant rural black folk, both men and women. However, it is striking how often black women were the objects of scrutiny in his stories about spreading disease to whites.

Consider the moral of the following tale, one of many told to black and white audiences. Moton, in his capacity as head of the Negro Organization Society, presented it to an audience one evening during a black health campaign in an attempt to appeal to whites:

> There was a colored woman in Atlanta who had been washing for a white family for 20 years. She had three grandchildren. She took the clothes home one Friday afternoon, and the mistress of the house met her and said, "Aunt Hannah, you mustn't come into the house, my little grandchild has scarlet fever, so leave the clothes out on the porch. I do not want your grandchildren to get the fever." Aunt Hannah said, "Laws, Honey, don't you worry about having scarlet fever. I have three grandchildren, and the last one is peeling now."[28]

Such tales sent a warning that white families paid the price for black women's ignorance. Dr. Algernon Jackson, a black doctor and instructor at Howard University, used the same plot in a story about Amanda, a black washerwoman, and the measles.[29] In each case the black laundress unwittingly transmitted scarlet fever (or measles) to the white family, even as the white mistress tried to protect the health of the black woman's family.

Moton considered such scare stories an effective way to raise white interest in black health, especially among women. Moton reported to a black audience that the Negro Organization Society of Virginia received widespread white cooperation for its black health campaigns because white people accepted the argument that white lives were at risk. "Because if we die, they die," explained Moton, "if we get diseased, they will get diseased, and they know it."[30]

The fear that germs did not respect the color line also appeared in the white southern press in a parallel form. Early in the century, an editorial in an Atlanta newspaper advised that despite segregation, white people were not safe from disease in black neighborhoods

> Because from that segregated district negro nurses would still emerge from diseased homes, to come into our homes and hold our children in their arms; negro cooks would still bring bacilli from the segregated district into the homes of the poor and the rich white Atlantan; negro chauffeurs, negro butlers, negro laborers would come from within the pale and scatter disease.[31]

According to the author, "to purge the negro of disease is not so much a kindness to the negro himself as it is a matter of sheer self-preservation to the white man."[32]

When Washington and Moton invoked their warnings about the risks white people faced from black illness, they were motivated by different political goals than the white press. They used concern for white health as a way to expose the contradictions and hypocrisy of segregation in the South and improve conditions for African Americans. They also preached these morality tales to black audiences, perhaps believing that the stories served as valuable forms of health education, even if delivered at the expense of reinforcing stereotypes about black women.

Why did black women carry the burdens of sickness in southern society? Black women may have been the focus of these stories because they came in frequent, intimate contact with white people in their capacity as workers. Often the only employment open to black women was domestic work in white homes, where employers expected them to cook, clean, and care for children. Furthermore, women were often the targets of health education campaigns because in their homes they held the main responsibility for the health of their families. To a great extent, then, black women carried the burdens of sickness because of the gendered division of household labor and the stratification of the labor market along racial and gender lines.

Consider the mixed messages of blame and black female agency contained in the following lecture by Washington. He painted a picture of the black woman worker that highlighted both the dangers of black ignorance and the importance of black labor. He told an audience of the Negro Organization Society of Virginia in 1914:

> When food is being prepared, the Negro touches the white man's life; when food is being served, the Negro woman touches the white man's life; when children are being nursed, the Negro woman touches the white man's life; when clothes are being laundered, the Negro woman touches the white man's life. It is mighty important, in the interest of our race as well as in the interest of the white race, that the Negro woman be taught cleanliness and the laws of health. Disease draws no color line.[33]

His message could be read in several ways. Washington explicitly indicated the need for health education for black women, but he also offered an implicit reminder of how dependent white people were on black women's labor. His emphasis on the significant impact of black women on white lives may have been an empowering message for black audiences and a reminder to whites of the importance of black Americans to southern society.

Calling on the State: Public Servants and Black Health Promotion

Washington only lived long enough to witness the first observance of National Negro Health Week, although he believed in the importance of the health campaign and tried to ensure its continuation. Shortly before his death in November 1915, Washington wrote to Anson Phelps Stokes to secure funding for the next year's health week.[34] However, without Washington's leadership the campaign was abandoned at first and no health week call went out from Tuskegee Institute in 1916. A year later, members of the National Negro Business League revived black health week. When league member and club woman Nannie Helen Burroughs contacted Washington's former secretary and fellow league member Emmett Scott at Tuskegee with some ideas for health week, Scott was eager to hear her suggestions. "We must keep the movement alive," he agreed, "not for the sake of the Business League so much as for the sake of this race of ours."[35]

Washington's successor Robert Moton struggled to establish his own place in the shadow of the Tuskegee "wizard." Moton attempted to carry out Washington's health program despite such interruptions as World War I and the deadly worldwide influenza epidemic of 1918–19.[36] By the early 1920s, Moton and Work concluded that private organizing efforts were not enough to make the kinds of larger changes needed to improve black health conditions. Although Tuskegee's leaders did not abandon community health campaigns, they turned increasingly to the state for assistance.

NATIONAL NEGRO HEALTH WEEK PLANNING COMMITTEE

Moton's first step toward broadening responsibility and establishing organizational support for the black health week program was to develop a formal structure of annual planning meetings to set policy. Beginning in 1921, Moton invited representatives from national organizations, particularly those interested in health and social welfare, to attend meetings held during the Annual Tuskegee Negro Conferences. Moton recruited black and white leaders in the belief that interracial cooperation would help to improve black access to existing services from government and private organizations.

Throughout the 1920s several black and white organizations joined Tuskegee in the effort to improve black health. Eight national black organizations sent representatives to the planning meetings and promoted black health week among their membership, including the National Association

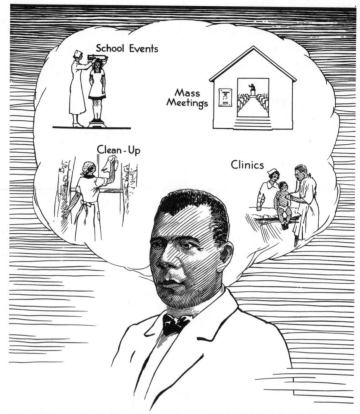

Booker T. Washington - A Man of Vision - Organized National Negro Health Week, 1915
" WHERE THERE IS NO VISION, THE PEOPLE PERISH / "

Figure 1. National Negro Health Week poster honoring Booker T. Washington. Courtesy of the National Archives, Washington, D.C.

for Teachers in Colored Schools and the National Association of Colored Graduate Nurses, with the NAACP notable for its absence.[37] The National Urban League and its local chapters put a tremendous amount of time and resources into the health week movement from the very beginning.[38] Furthermore, fifteen white organizations, such as the American Red Cross and the National Tuberculosis Association, sent representatives each year.[39] Most of the twenty to forty representatives at the annual planning meetings were black men, including Monroe Work and Robert Moton. For example, in 1927 among those attending were twenty black men, eight black women, seven white women, and three white men.[40]

Throughout the 1920s the topics at health week planning meetings began to extend beyond Negro Health Week to include a wide variety of issues. Participants discussed the need to promote birth and death registration of African Americans, encourage studies about the diseases of black people, expand training and opportunities for black physicians and nurses, encourage periodic physical examinations, improve urban housing conditions, and increase health care facilities in rural and urban areas. Participants also recommended that government representatives be asked to sit on health week planning committees at the community level.[41] Finally, one of the first committee decisions was to honor Booker T. Washington as founder of National Negro Health Week by celebrating it each year on April 5, his birthday (see Figure 1).[42]

Committee members set two main goals: (1) to expand health week activities into a year-round black public health campaign, and (2) to encourage the federal government to take over responsibility for organizing black public health work. One way to achieve this expansion was for the USPHS to sponsor the National Negro Health Week program and, in the words of Work, "thereby insure its permanence."[43]

LOBBYING GOVERNMENT POLICYMAKERS

Robert Moton and Monroe Work wanted government support to lend legitimacy to their health efforts. They managed to convince officials at the USPHS to provide official government endorsement of National Negro Health Week and access to government resources.[44] In 1921 Moton requested endorsement from U.S. Surgeon General Hugh Cumming, head of the USPHS, in order to pressure public health officers across the country to assist with black health week campaigns. Cumming agreed and offered government printing facilities to publish a health week bulletin for health education and publicity purposes. The bulletins initially provided information about specific diseases, but gradually they focused more on explaining how to organize a health week program, such as creating a home hygiene day on Monday, community sanitation day on Tuesday, children's health day on Wednesday, and so on. Government facilities printed the bulletin every year after 1921, although apparently Tuskegee continued to cover most of the cost, which amounted to about $550 each year.[45] Beginning in 1925, Moton and Work also convinced the Surgeon General to permit the planning committee to meet at the USPHS every fall. These provisions indicate the federal government was willing to play a role, albeit a minor one, in support of black health promotion.[46]

Black leaders tried several approaches to bringing black health needs to the attention of local and national health policymakers. A major concern was to persuade government health agencies to hire black personnel.[47] A steady stream of correspondence from Tuskegee Institute urged agencies to hire black health workers. In 1923 Moton suggested to Assistant Surgeon General Thomas Parran that the USPHS follow the lead of the U.S. Department of Agriculture, which employed several hundred black men and women agents in the South through the Extension Service.[48] That same year National Urban League leader Jesse O. Thomas, a 1911 graduate of Tuskegee Institute, suggested to Moton that black leaders embark on a careful, sustained push for state-level health appointments of African Americans to parallel the hiring of black assistant superintendents of education. "I do not believe we are going to ever arrive unless we increase our personnel in this whole health effort," he explained.[49] Black leaders believed that hiring black health professionals was one way to expand health week into year-round activity.

The development of permanent black health councils in communities across the nation was another way to expand beyond the limitations of a once-a-year focus on black health. Indeed, this idea was first proposed at the 1921 health week planning meeting. By 1926 many of the Negro Health Week committees at the local level had developed into permanent health councils. Such councils provided the opportunity for community monitoring of black health conditions. Thomas suggested to Moton that every local committee contact "the State, County and Municipal Boards of Health with a view of calling specific attention to certain unsanitary and unwholesome conditions effecting [sic] the Negro in particular and the whole people in general."[50]

Despite their concern for health reform, black health activists did not offer an explicit critique of a profit-oriented health care system. In the United States, unlike most other industrialized nations, no publicly funded health care system developed in the twentieth century, in part because of the resistance of the white medical profession to "socialized medicine."[51] However, by the 1920s black activists insisted that the state had an obligation to meet the health needs of all its citizens. Moton argued that "in the last analysis, it is the state's business to see to the people's health."[52] Work echoed this sentiment, stating that the preservation of health "was a public matter and that it was the duty of public health agencies, Municipal, State and National to take the lead."[53]

Spreading the Gospel of Health and Cleanliness: White Officials, Black Professionals, and Community Women

By the late 1920s, National Negro Health Week altered, if ever so slightly, the focus of public health policy and the practice of public health work. It helped put black health on the government's public health agenda, even if only to safeguard the health of whites. Leaders at Tuskegee Institute saw increasing evidence that white health officials, black professionals, and community women were interested in improving black health conditions.

Campaigns in communities across the South and into the North focused on health education, individual hygiene, and environmental sanitation, with special emphasis on housing conditions. Health reformers spoke of "spreading the gospel of health" to black America, a phrase used throughout the early twentieth century to refer to messages about the laws of health. For example, in 1929 Bernice Scott from Horsehead, New York, contacted Tuskegee Institute about her interest in the Negro Health Week campaign. "I would like to include your program on my visits to the towns and city in spreading the gospel of health to the race people in this western part of New York state as I am doing social health work."[54]

"Cleanliness" was the most important focus of early health week activity, and in a sense it honored the work that women did. By 1900 personal and household cleanliness had become a habit of the American middle class and a major message of reformers who worked among the poor.[55] Black health campaigns combined the disease-prevention strategies of the sanitation movement of the nineteenth century, with its focus on cleaning up the environment, and the new public health tactics of the early twentieth century, with their attention to personal hygiene and germs.[56] Black health projects incorporated a commitment to racial uplift and pride through programs geared toward cleaning up and beautifying premises; removing trash and garbage; whitewashing or painting homes, schools, and churches; planting gardens; and generally removing any "symptoms of slovenliness." As one journalist reported, through health week activities "good housewives have pronounced the death penalty on germs."[57]

Community health activists equated health with cleanliness and cleanliness with respectability. Club women in particular placed great emphasis on creating attractive home surroundings. A woman from Jackson, Mississippi, explained that club women wanted black neighborhoods to be as nice as any other sections of town, and she emphasized that "there is no reason why a stranger coming into Jackson should be able to identify a neighborhood as being the home of Negroes by sagging fences, broken window panes, dirty premises, lack of sidewalks, and dusty streets."[58] In 1930 in Nashville, Tennessee, Negro Health Week focused on clean-up work. Black women from twenty-five women's clubs inspected fourteen of the "most backward areas of the city" and urged the "housewives" to clean up the premises. The city health department also inspected barber shops, beauty parlors, meat shops, grocery stores, restaurants, and theaters in black neighborhoods for adequate sanitation. When health week ended, the hundred black women and men of the health week committee created a permanent Negro Health Council to continue their health activities.[59]

The moral dimension of cleanliness affected black activists' racial uplift work. National Baptist leader, club woman, and educator Nannie Helen Burroughs employed the metaphor of "cleanliness" as a guiding motto for the National Training School for Women and Girls, which she established in 1909 in Washington, D.C. She taught her students to follow "the three B's — the Bible, the bath, the broom: clean life, clean body, clean home."[60] Even the 1905 "Declaration of Principles" from the Niagara Movement included the following: "We plead for health — for an opportunity to live in decent houses and localities, for a chance to rear our children in physical and moral cleanliness."[61]

The thousands of health week reports sent to Tuskegee Institute by local health week committees during the 1920s attest to the widespread observance of National Negro Health Week. Tuskegee leaders enticed communities to submit reports describing their local campaigns by turning submissions into entries for an annual health week contest. A variety of volunteers, including Alice Dunbar-Nelson, a black teacher and writer from Delaware, and Jessie Fauset, a black novelist from New York, served as judges for these contests.[62] In 1917 the National Clean-Up and Paint-Up Campaign Bureau began providing trophies for the best health week observances as judged by the reports. This organization, supported by paint and varnish manufacturers, operated under the slogan: "Cleanliness, thrift, and civic pride — the essentials for homes and towns beautiful."[63]

Health week activities were even more widespread than such reports indicated because many communities, perhaps most, never bothered to send in descriptions of their health campaigns. For example, in 1929 Tuskegee received only 46 formal health week reports: seven from cities over 100,000, twelve from cities under 100,000, and twenty-seven from rural districts.[64] Yet, Tuskegee received notices of health week observances from 470 communities that year, and certainly many places did not even bother to send a notice.[65] Ruth Henderson of the American Red Cross pointed out that it was too difficult for volunteers to write up the details.[66] F. Rivers Barnwell, director of black health work for the Texas Public Health Association, wrote to Work: "You have often heard me say that I am not ashamed of the work done by the Texas group during the WEEK but they just fall down on the making of their reports."[67] It remains, then, extremely difficult to estimate the number of communities that participated in National Negro Health Week during the 1920s, but hundreds, perhaps thousands, did.

Black leaders tried to link black health week activity to existing government health programs, including the work of state boards of health and the health education work for mothers and babies of the U.S. Children's Bureau. In 1922 Moton contacted Grace Abbott, head of the Children's Bureau, and explained that "as in previous years we are asking your cooperation in this effort for health improvement. Whatever you may do to call this matter to the attention of the general public and also to those under your supervision will be greatly appreciated."[68] In 1925 Alabama state health officer Dr. S. W. Welch offered his endorsement when he wrote to all southern state health officers asking them to inform their health workers about Negro Health Week.[69] The following year Assistant Surgeon General W. F. Draper wrote to the state health officers of twenty states and received assurances that they would promote black health week. Assistant Surgeon General C. C. Pierce reported at a health week planning meeting, no doubt with some exaggeration, that "all of the state boards of health, and the city health departments are in sympathy to advance the idea of public health among negroes."[70]

INTERRACIAL COOPERATION: WHITE EFFORTS FOR BLACK HEALTH
Each year Tuskegee Institute received hundreds of letters requesting National Negro Health Week information not only from black teachers, ministers, doctors, nurses, and club women but also from a surprising number of white health officials. Many individual white health workers responded positively to appeals for black health programs. This interest was especially evident during the 1920s, the decade of a southern interracial movement.[71] For example, in 1929 when Tuskegee Institute contacted Dr. C. W. Garrison, state health officer of Arkansas, about promoting Negro Health Week, he responded: "I am pleased to advise that this office has already

ordered bulletins and posters."[72] In 1929 J. T. Irby, the white medical director of Crittenden County Health Department in Arkansas, requested that
Tuskegee send him health literature

> available for distribution among civic and other organizations of your people
> in my county. I am anxious to get the people of the various communities
> interested in this health movement as early as possible. Last year during health
> week some very good work was done in several places in this county and this
> year we hope to accomplish much more.[73]

White health officers could be important allies for black health work.

Some white women actively supported National Negro Health Week
campaigns in their roles as professionals and community workers. In War-
rensburg, Missouri, a white county nurse who received a copy of a health
week bulletin made the effort to write to Tuskegee to apologize that the
nursing service, which had been in the county a year, had "not done very
much health work among the negroes," but that she was eager to assist
the black communities with their health week plans.[74] When Mrs. W. L.
Thompson, superintendent of social services in Wrightsville, Georgia,
wrote to Tuskegee requesting health information to help black people in
her town, Moton responded with much encouragement. He suggested that
she initiate black health week activities, stating: "You will be interested to
know that in a number of communities in the South White Women's Clubs
are taking the lead in this effort for the Health Improvement of the Colored
people."[75] Public health work appealed to women's interests in community
improvement. White women's cooperation in black health work may have
been motivated in part by fears that "germs know no color line," but health
promotion was consistent with women's ongoing involvement in social
welfare activity.

Moton became convinced that health work improved race relations.
"Health work," he noted, "has been found to be one of the most effective
methods of bringing the two races together on a platform of mutual confidence and respect and with a mutual desire to help."[76] Indeed, the reports of
Negro Health Week campaigns in several cities indicated that black health
week organizers believed that some degree of interracial health work was
possible.

Evidence of white cooperation was welcomed by African Americans in
an era of ongoing racial tensions. For instance, in 1927 in Louisville, Kentucky, Negro Health Week organizers represented their accomplishments
in terms of interracial cooperation. A local chapter of the Young Men's

Christian Association (YMCA) organized the black health week under the leadership of Dr. James Bond, director of the Interracial Commission of the black division of the YMCA for the state of Kentucky. In his health week report, Bond explained that "it is impossible of course in a report like this to get over entirely the fine spirit of Interracial cooperation that characterized the campaign both in Louisville and throughout the state." He continued: "The by-product of interracial good will and cooperation was probably as valuable an asset as the health work messages themselves."[77]

An interracial component was also central to the black health week observance in Cincinnati, Ohio. In 1927 the Negro Civic Welfare Association, a department of the Community Chest and Council of Social Agencies, organized Negro Health Week. Eighteen community organizations assisted with the health campaign, and black and white men and women, Christians and Jews, sat on the executive committee. Members of a Jewish temple provided their building for the opening and closing mass meetings, and W. E. B. Du Bois gave an address at the opening event. Health week activities included films, distribution of literature, baby clinics, vaccination programs, and school lectures. Health week supporters visited nearly six hundred homes in a house-to-house health education campaign. Organizers also convinced the city health department to inspect shops and restaurants in the black district of the city, and "nine landlords owning property in the Negro district cooperated by making structural repairs and assisting in the removal of rubbish."[78] Negro Health Week campaigns could effectively promote cooperation across racial lines, which many saw as a key to black advancement.

MAKING THE CONNECTION: BLACK WOMEN'S COMMUNITY HEALTH WORK

Black women professionals and community workers used the observance of National Negro Health Week to make claims for black entitlement to a share of community resources. They struggled to bring together black residents and government health services through endless fund-raising and lobbying. Black nurses, teachers, Jeanes Supervisors (black supervisors of teachers), home demonstration agents, and club women predominated in health education and public health work at the community level.[79] They worked with local chapters of national black and white organizations to sponsor black health week, hire black personnel in health departments, and establish clinics for African Americans.[80] From Mississippi to New York to Washington state, black women promoted public health work.[81]

Much of black women's community health activity was directed at soliciting funds because black organizations were usually plagued by a shortage of money. In order to supplement their meagre funds, health week organizers sought financial assistance from local governments and charity associations. The Community Chest, a philanthropic organization that dispersed funds to worthy city projects, was often a target. For example, a black woman in the state of Washington reported to Tuskegee Institute that Seattle's health week organizers had sought to "secure our rightful share from the organizations which work for social betterment, the Welfare League and the Community Chest."[82]

Black women's efforts increased the possibility that black people would participate in public health programs. The black women who organized the Negro Health Week campaign in Seattle chose to focus on the health needs of black children and then establish city services to meet those needs. Their strategy was to develop contact with every black child in the area. Ten women each took charge of a city district and obtained the names and addresses of all black children. The women of the health week committee then provided free transportation to the clinics in order to ensure a high turnout. Mrs. Gordon Carter, a black woman who chaired the health week committee, reported that a nurse from Seattle's Department of Child Hygiene provided free physical examinations for preschool children at the black branch of the Young Women's Christian Association (YWCA). The committee used the information gained from the clinic "as a factual basis for determining the social service activity needed by our children," according to Carter. She explained that the data gathered assisted the women in dealing with the local government and allowed them to "present any claim for service with a degree of accuracy."[83]

A significant amount of black women's health activity centered on creating community health clinics because of the inadequate number of health facilities available to black people, especially the poor. For example, in Georgia the Savannah Federation of Colored Women's Clubs, representing over a hundred separate clubs, established the Cuyler Children's Free Clinic. Volunteers staffed the clinic, which was under the full control and financial responsibility of the federated women's clubs. Club women convinced black and white physicians to donate medical services, and they lobbied city and county commissioners to cover the costs of the clinic and the salary of a nurse. Throughout the 1920s and into the 1930s the clinic provided free health care to about four hundred poor children each month and a Tuesday clinic to test for syphilis in adults, mostly domestics, laborers, and the unemployed.[84]

Permanent health councils, which among other things promoted Negro Health Week observances, grew out of black women's participation in community health education programs. Black women in Boston and Detroit, for example, created their own health councils after graduating from city health education courses. In 1929 in Boston, forty black women ranging in age from twenty to sixty formed a Health Guild in the Boston Tuberculosis Association to promote health education in black neighborhoods.[85] A year later in Detroit, two hundred black women formed the Daniel Hale Williams' Health Guild. This health organization, named after the famous black surgeon and founder of Chicago's Provident Hospital, organized an observance of Negro Health Week by soliciting assistance from the city department of health, black physicians, teachers, and ministers. The Health Guild members created a number of projects for Negro Health Week, including an eight-week health clinic held in black churches that immunized over 5,000 children against diphtheria. The members divided the city into fourteen districts, each with a chair and twenty assistants, to arrange health education lectures and health examinations at local black schools, churches, and women's clubs. Finally, they oversaw neighborhood clean-up campaigns and visited every home in their district, handing out literature on family health to mothers.[86]

In many communities, health week organizers secured city services that local governments had not previously extended to black neighborhoods. For example, in Waco, Texas, the Volunteer Health League procured the assistance of the local health department, which then "furnished trash trucks to take away all trash." According to Mrs. R. V. Estelle, the League next planned to establish a free clinic, playgrounds, and provisions for better drainage and lighting in black neighborhoods, as well as secure a black truant officer, school nurse, county nurse, and policewoman.[87]

Black communities repeatedly faced the burden of convincing government officials that black health could, and should, be improved. They had to counter white beliefs about apathy among poor black people and demonstrate that the poor cared enough about their health to warrant government service, including the appointment of health officers. Thomasville, a small rural black community in Alabama, celebrated health week with a health meeting one night at the First Baptist Church and another at the Methodist Church. At the closing meeting the people attending drew up a petition requesting a health officer be appointed to their community. Mrs. M. N. Dickinson, president of the county Parent-Teachers Association and principal of the Marvin District School, chaired the nine-member health week committee. Dickinson wrote to Tuskegee Institute for information about how her community could go about getting a health officer "to look after the health of school children, and sanitary conditions of the town." Work responded to her inquiry by advising her to "consult the Probate Judge and have a conference with some of the leading Physicians in your community along with some influential citizens and discuss this matter carefully." He told her that if all agreed that the health officer is needed, she could file an application with the Alabama Department of Health.[88]

Black women played a prominent role in one of the largest National Negro Health Week campaigns of the decade, which took place in Chicago. In 1929 forty community organizations joined with the black Cook County Physicians' Association to put on a three-week health campaign. Chicago's forty-two-page health week report provides evidence of the type of massive mobilization it was possible to achieve when many segments of a community united toward a common goal. One of the campaign's features was the extensive participation of women on planning committees and in leadership roles. These women, in turn, increased the involvement of community-based organizations and local residents. A variety of organizations supported Chicago's health project, including black women's clubs, local black nurses' associations, the Douglas League of Women Voters, the Phyllis Wheatley Association, the South Side Settlement House, and the NAACP.[89] According to one participant, the campaign was "without a doubt one of the most intensive campaigns of its kind ever conducted in the city of Chicago."[90]

Chicago's health week report singled out two black women for their contributions to the success of the year's health week, which reached 50,000 people on a budget of $115. Maude A. Lawrence, a member of the Chicago Urban League, and Isabel Lawson, a member of the Chicago YWCA, succeeded in rounding up twice as many organizations to participate in the health campaign in 1929 as there were the year before.[91] They both served on several committees, including the committee to arrange for speakers and the committee to select health topics, the second of which chose to focus on respiratory diseases, heart disease, cancer, venereal disease, rickets, nursing care, and dental disorders.

A number of black people, especially health professionals and community women, donated their time to the health campaign. The committee on speakers sent out over 250 letters to dentists, physicians, and nurses to arrange for volunteers and ended up with health presentations by forty-five physicians, thirty-three dentists, and seven nurses. These volunteers gave talks to eleven fraternal groups, twenty-two women's clubs, thirteen industrial groups, nineteen high schools, twenty-two grammar schools, and twenty-nine churches.[92] Approximately sixty African Americans sat on twelve planning committees. About half the committee members were women and half were male doctors. Four black women doctors participated, including Dr. Mary F. Waring, a leader in the National Association of Colored Women.[93]

Chicago's health campaign went beyond public educational programs to provide dental and medical clinics, a trend that increased in the following decades. In addition to the health talks, health pageant, baby contest, and presentations of twenty-six different health films borrowed from the Illinois Board of Health, the health campaign also offered free clinics in the evenings.[94] The health report noted that "interest of the public in the periodic examination exceeded our most sanguine expectations." Over 250 women and men received free dental examinations from twenty dentists who worked four-hour shifts. Over three hundred people, most likely working class, sent in their applications for appointments at the medical clinic, and the clinic staff members were surprised when as many as 275 of these people showed up. Despite public perceptions of African Americans as a diseased population, about 35 percent of those seen by the staff were in perfect health, and many of the remainder had only minor health problems. Some of the people exhibited heart disease or high blood pressure, but there were almost no cases of tuberculosis, and only five of the 171 people given Wassermann tests to check for venereal disease tested positive.[95]

Here, in the administration of health week, women's efforts were most apparent. In these clinics, held during the evening, most of the support staff were women. Some twenty-five nurses assisted dentists and physicians, while twenty-four laywomen distributed in the community applications for clinic appointments, contacted patients with appointment times, and acted as scribes for the physicians and dentists during examinations. Patients gave a complete history, describing their living and working conditions, before each medical examination.

As with all public health work, there were limitations to Chicago's health week clinic provisions. Staff notified all patients of the findings from medical examinations, but if doctors detected any problems they told people to consult their family physician — advice that rested on the faulty assumption that all patients could afford one. Medical staff at these clinics gave no treatments or prescriptions, thus limiting their services only to detection of disease and leaving treatment to private physicians.[96] Although it is likely that even this was more health care attention than many people had received previously, the situation points out that health activists were unable or unwilling to challenge the boundaries between private practice and public health.

Assessing the Impact of National Negro Health Week to 1930

Despite the shortage of funds to finance a full-time coordinator for the national promotion of Negro Health Week, the effort under Tuskegee Institute from 1915 to 1930 reached millions of African Americans. In 1929 Work declared that the health week movement had grown so much that "it can be regarded as an institution."[97] In 1930 Tuskegee Institute provided figures, no doubt produced by Work, drawn from correspondence, news-clippings, and formal health week reports, of the number of communities observing National Negro Health Week. The figures indicated that there were health week programs in several hundred communities each year from 1925 to 1930. However, because most communities did not notify Tuskegee of their programs, Work concluded that at least 2,500 communities celebrated health week annually. On average, thirty-two states held campaigns each year, ranging from California to Wisconsin to Mississippi, with southern states most represented. Activity even spread beyond the United States to Montreal, Canada, and British colonies in West Africa.[98]

In addition to this evidence of interest in health week, Tuskegee leaders believed that the campaign improved black health. In 1924 Work reported that since the beginning of the campaign, the black death rate dropped from 23 deaths per 1,000 people to 15, and black life expectancy increased from thirty-five to forty years. "This means," he explained, "that in the 10 years since National Negro Health Week was established, the lifespan of Negroes of the United States has been increased 5 years. This is a great achievement."[99] Many factors contributed to such signs of improvement, but public health work was certainly among them.

For Moton and Work, the greatest impact on black health conditions would come when the federal government took responsibility for the health of all citizens. They wanted the USPHS to take over National Negro Health Week and make it into a year-round program under the supervision of medical experts. By the end of the decade they began to see signs that their lobbying would pay off: in 1929 the national health week planning committee passed a resolution to make National Negro Health Week into "a year-round, full-time, self-perpetuating movement in order that there might be a clearing-house for coordination of the several health activities" supporting black health improvement. Surgeon General Cumming endorsed the decision to place the movement "upon a more substantial basis. As now conducted the work is rather sporadic and not as continuous as it should be."[100]

In the early 1930s the federal government responded to the call from black health leaders for formal support of National Negro Health Week when the USPHS, with financial assistance from the Rosenwald Fund, took over responsibility. The Rosenwald Fund was a private philanthropic foundation established by Julius Rosenwald, owner of the Sears Department Store Company and a trustee of Tuskegee Institute. This fund, which Booker T. Washington had encouraged Rosenwald to establish in 1912, now kept Washington's movement afloat.[101]

Instead of being the cooptation of a black-led project, black leaders wanted the USPHS to take over the campaign. It pleased Moton and Work to relinquish Tuskegee's responsibility for the black health week program and see it turned into an official, government-sponsored black health movement. Moton told Cumming "that the time has come when it should be taken over by agencies primarily interested in health improvement and able to furnish the expert direction necessary to its further development."[102] Having met their major goals during the 1920s, black leaders remained hopeful that their achievements would bring about the expansion of opportunities for black health workers, the creation of ever more health institutions, and the eventual development of a health care system with no color line.

Finally, it is important to recognize the critical political dimensions of black efforts to spread the gospel of health. Supporters of National Negro Health Week not only performed social service work when they created health programs previously unavailable to most African Americans, they also engaged in political activity to extend black rights when they lobbied local governments and private organizations. In defending black entitlement to existing public provisions, African Americans challenged the inequality of the racially segregated health care system.

3. A New Deal for Black Health
Community Activism and the
Office of Negro Health Work

The establishment of the Office of Negro Health Work during the New Deal era marked a milestone in the history of American public health. It was the first time since the Freedmen's Bureau of the post-Civil War era that the federal government institutionalized black health work within the federal bureaucracy. In 1932 the lobbying efforts of black leaders paid off, and the United States Public Health Service (USPHS) opened the Office of Negro Health Work as a clearinghouse for black health activity and as headquarters for the National Negro Health Week campaign, which became a year-round effort called the National Negro Health Movement.

After 1920 the history of black public health work is best understood by examining the interaction of government and private initiatives. In particular, the Great Depression of the 1930s accelerated federal government involvement in social welfare, including black health.[1] President Franklin D. Roosevelt inaugurated the New Deal to ease the massive socioeconomic crisis of the Depression; as a result the locus of control over public health issues shifted from the states to the federal government. In line with other New Deal programs of the 1930s, the work of the USPHS reached into the South and attempted to override some of the resistance to the extension of state services to black people. Even though racism and segregation restricted black access to most, if not all, New Deal programs, the federal government provided more health benefits to African Americans than southern state governments had provided.[2]

Ultimately, the federal government merely supplemented the ongoing voluntary labor of African Americans, who created their own "new deal" for black health through community activism. Repeatedly, grassroots community efforts stimulated and facilitated the public health work of city and county governments.[3] Yet, despite this advocacy work at the local and national level, African Americans were not a political priority for government officials. If federal activity reached black communities, it invariably rested on a foundation of black health programs put into place by middle-class black activists well before the New Deal. Although inroads were made, the USPHS and local health departments failed to demonstrate a serious commitment to black health improvement and thus to black rights. Without community activism, much of it carried out by black women, public health work simply would not have reached most black communities.

Throughout the twentieth century, black public health work has been gendered. For example, black men, many of them doctors, were prominent at the national level in the establishment of the National Negro Health Movement and the Office of Negro Health Work. But it would be wrong to characterize this effort as simply male-dominated and doctor-controlled because women, most of whom were layworkers, were the ones who shaped the implementation of health policy. Black women's contributions were greatest at the local level, where their ability to mobilize community participation was vital to the success of black health programs and the expansion of health week into a mass movement. As family and community caretakers, women provided the personal contact between the health programs and the targets of health reform. The success of public health activity cannot be measured only by the development of policy, medicine, and government activity without attention also to administration, nursing, and laywomen's volunteer labor.

Private Practice and Public Health Policy: Black Doctors and the Federal Government

The creation of the Office of Negro Health Work is evidence of the impact, albeit limited, of black health activism on the federal government. For a decade black activists had argued for black entitlement to federal government services. Meanwhile the National Medical Association (NMA), the national black medical organization, had argued for the employment of black personnel within the USPHS. The development of the Office of Negro Health Work, under the direction of black health education specialist Dr. Roscoe C. Brown, was a sign of success. Although most of the official records of this government office, as well as Brown's personal papers, were lost or destroyed, there is extensive reference to the work of Brown and the Office of Negro Health Work in other government records and black medical sources.[4]

Dr. Roscoe C. Brown and the USPHS

Dr. Roscoe C. Brown (1884–1962), who served as the liaison between the USPHS and black communities, was one of the most prominent black public health leaders of the twentieth century. He was the sole black official in the USPHS during the 1930s and was also the only public health official in the "Black Cabinet" of President Roosevelt's administration. Throughout his life Brown remained diligent in his efforts to bring black health needs to the attention of the nation. Indeed, it is a testimony to the efforts of public health workers like Brown that the topic of black health achieved such national visibility that in 1940 *Time* magazine reported that Negro health was the nation's "No. 1 public health problem."[5]

Brown became involved in public health work early in his career. Born in Washington, D.C., he earned a dental degree in 1906 from Howard University Dental School, practiced dentistry for nearly a decade, and then turned his full attention to public health work.[6] During the 1910s he lived in Richmond, Virginia, and taught hygiene and sanitation at Richmond Hospital, served as a visiting dentist at the St. Francis de Sales Institute, and assisted the Negro Organization Society of Virginia. He also became an active member of the NMA and the National Dental Association.[7]

Brown was one of a select few black professionals hired by the USPHS during World War I when the government became interested in the prevention of venereal disease.[8] In 1919 the recently established Division of Venereal Disease in the USPHS hired him to provide health education for African Americans, following his term in field service work for the Office of the Surgeon General of the Army the year before. Brown had two black assistants, Dr. Ralph Stewart and Walter J. Hughes, and together they prepared pamphlets and public lectures about venereal disease and treatments. They also created educational exhibits, including "Keeping Fit" for black boys and "Youth and Life" for black girls.[9] In the 1920s Brown and Stewart continued to spread the word to black communities, including Tuskegee Institute, about the dangers of venereal disease and the importance of sex education, and they promoted education about venereal diseases as part of National Negro Health Week observances. According to the head of the division, "we thought it was not wise to put out a program devoted entirely to one phase of preventive medicine, so we made it a broad disease prevention program in which venereal diseases were given a place."[10] No doubt the stigma associated with venereal disease led the division to couch its work in general public health terms. Brown worked for the USPHS until 1923, when loss of funding and the pressure of a "decentralization" policy forced him to quit, as conservatives reasserted states' rights in the post-war period. According to Brown, this move spelled disaster because without federal control over health work in the states, black public health efforts were doomed.[11]

Although Brown was no longer a full-time employee of the USPHS, he maintained his affiliation on an informal basis throughout the decade. He continued to work as a lecturer and special consultant for the USPHS, even representing the federal government at National Negro Health Week planning meetings. He went out on the lecture circuit and promoted observances of Negro Health Week throughout the South. In 1923, for example, he spent two weeks in Texas promoting black health for the Texas Public Health Association, and in 1927 he traveled for several weeks, presenting thirty-four lectures on venereal disease and general health to 14,000 people for Negro Health Week in North Carolina, Tennessee, Georgia, and Alabama.[12]

Even when Brown was not a full-time employee, he still had an impact on federal health policy. In the late 1920s he convinced U.S. Surgeon General Hugh Cumming to authorize the first study on black mortality by the federal government. Brown used the old refrain about disease and the color line to argue for the investigation. "You know of course, that this is not only a protective service for our group," he pointed out, "but also a means of security for all people in view of the fact that health and disease alike have an interdependence affecting both groups." Cumming endorsed the study but cautioned Brown that "other important studies" had priority. Two years later the USPHS finally completed the research and published the health bulletin "Mortality Among Negroes in the United States."[13] This accomplishment was a result of Brown's lobbying efforts and one of the many ways that black activists influenced federal health work.

Public Health and the National Medical Association

The black and white medical professions had an ambiguous relationship to the field of public health. Public health work remained a relatively low priority for organized medicine, leading a few doctors to berate their fellow practitioners for ignoring public needs. Public health work took a back seat for most doctors because of the curative focus of twentieth-century American medicine in general and because in the United States medicine operated according to the profit motive like any other business. However, some black and white doctors were very active in public health reform and became leaders of public health movements. The black and white medical professions did not forsake public health concerns, but the same few doctors did most of the work.[14]

Given this context, it is not surprising that most black male physicians paid more attention to their private practices than to public health activity.[15] Yet, caution is warranted in constructing generalizations that characterize black physicians this way until further research permits comparisons by race and gender among twentieth-century medical professionals. By and large, black doctors were very aware of the public health needs of black communities, but like most white doctors, public health projects were not their primary interest.

Although the NMA heartily endorsed National Negro Health Week efforts, presidents of the organization occasionally expressed concern that doctors did not do enough. In his presidential address in 1927 Dr. Carl Robert commended the public health activity led by Tuskegee Institute but noted:

> It is regrettable that they have not received the co-operation to which they are entitled from the medical profession. It is true that in scattered localities the response has been excellent, but the attitude of the medical men has varied from perfunctory participation to actual indifference.[16]

The NMA repeatedly reminded local medical societies to do their share in promoting Negro Health Week.[17]

Some black doctors, both physicians and dentists, may have felt too burdened by their efforts to establish and sustain private practices in the era of Jim Crow to participate in health week projects, even though they endorsed the work. By 1930 black medical institutions had produced some 3,700 black physicians, a sizable number but still far too few for the needs of black America.[18] Occasionally black doctors did address public needs but in their own private ways. For example, a southern black dentist who graduated from Howard University Dental School in 1917 led his own campaign to provide sufficient food and clothing to poor children in his community so they could attend school.[19] Other doctors may simply have had no interest in public health activity.

There were black doctors who volunteered for health week campaigns, although a few did not provide all they had promised. After the local black medical society in Birmingham, Alabama, took part in the city's health week program, a doctor commented that he was glad to see the men finally performing their duty to their community. As a result of this health week activity, the doctors formed a welfare committee within their medical society.[20] In Louisville, Kentucky, several doctors gave health lectures for Negro Health Week in churches, at eighteen black schools, and at meetings of the Young Women's Christian Association (YWCA) and of black club women. However, although doctors had agreed to give health lectures in over forty black churches on the Sunday that opened health week, health week organizers reported that "not all of the physicians kept their appointments. . . ." Health week organizers arranged for physicians to give talks in five factories, "but only one physician kept his appointment."[21] Perhaps unexpected demands took some doctors away from assisting with public health work even when they intended to help, while others may simply have concluded it was not worth the effort.

Despite the obstacles to doctors' participation, a few black dentists and physicians provided welcome assistance to health campaigns, especially women. Dr. Zenobia G. Gilpin, president of the Richmond Medical Society in Virginia, developed a program with the sponsorship of a local chapter of the Urban League and eighteen other organizations. Doctors, ministers, and many laywomen served on nine organizing committees. Doctors and church members gave health talks in each of the fifty-three black churches, reaching over 10,000 people. With no black hospital in the city, the health week focused on providing adult and children's clinics in the Baptist churches and a Presbyterian mission for Negroes. The female members of the committee on clinics organized subcommittees consisting of neighborhood women to help physicians and nurses at the clinics. The women tried to secure adult and child attendance through advertising campaigns and registering every neighborhood child on a card. About 150 adults and 180 children received medical examinations at the clinics. The members of one church even decided to make their building the site of a monthly clinic where black physicians could practice and black patients could receive treatment, unlike at the local white hospital.[22]

A few doctors even considered public health work an ideal opportunity to promote their profession as well as their own private practices.[23] Dr. Midian Othello Bousfield, who in 1934 became Director of Negro Health at the Julius Rosenwald Fund, helped organize an observance of black health week in Chicago in 1933, in which he emphasized the role of doctors. Bousfield encouraged Chicago's two-week health program in order to stimulate business for local black physicians and dentists. At health week lectures around the city, doctors provided audiences with lists of the names of members of the Cook County Physicians Association and the Lincoln Dental Society, and they explained that people could receive a free examination by visiting one of the doctors. Instead of holding health clinics at a central location, the health campaign sent people to the individual doctors' offices. The organizers hoped that by urging people to visit a doctor, the people would become regular customers, and the convenience for doctors would encourage the doctors to participate in the health campaigns.[24] Although the idea of promoting annual medical and dental examinations was consistent with the twentieth-century public health focus on individuals, such efforts appeared to be little more than free advertising for doctors in private practice.[25]

A few doctors argued that the black medical profession should assume the national leadership of the Negro Health Week movement. The issue of appropriate authority arose as early as 1915, several months before the first Negro Health Week observance. Dr. Algernon B. Jackson of Philadelphia, later director of the Department of Public Health at Howard University Medical School and a leader of the National Negro Health Movement, wrote Booker T. Washington that he thought the proposed health campaign should be under the control of the black medical association, not the control of laymen. Jackson advised Washington that at the very least the program "should be placed in the hands of a physician or committee of medical men who understand public health problems, or scientifically and practically it will be a failure."[26] It appears that Washington merely ignored Jackson's warning.

Yet, beginning in the late 1920s, doctors did play an increasing role in policy formulation for National Negro Health Week. For example, in 1927 Tuskegee leaders created an executive committee comprised of a few members of the annual health week planning committee. The executive committee included Dr. Roscoe C. Brown, Monroe Work, R. Maurice Ross of the National Urban League, Dr. James Bond of the Kentucky YMCA, and Dr. Algernon B. Jackson.[27] Over the years, more doctors were added to the committee.[28] The major black health issues of the day, and those discussed by the executive committee, were tuberculosis, venereal disease, infant mortality, and maternal mortality.[29] Yet, in 1932 the executive committee decided that although it would not discourage communities from addressing these issues, there were enough government and voluntary organizations focusing on them so that the black health movement could focus on a wide range of health issues.[30]

The prominence of black male doctors, all active members of the NMA, and the paucity of black women in the executive committee characterized national leadership patterns in the black health week movement over the next two decades. Indeed, the only black women ever to play a role in this decision-making body, even after the committee became a more informal fifteen-member advisory committee, were Mabel Keaton Staupers, a leader of the National Association of Colored Graduate Nurses who attended meetings from 1935 to 1945, and Modjeska Simpkins, a South Carolina health educator who attended from 1936 to 1941.[31]

The executive committee held the position that black doctors were best qualified to create health policy. In 1931 the committee concluded that even though local community organizations needed control over how they carried out the National Negro Health Movement, doctors were the rightful national leaders.[32] That same year, Brown drafted a five-year plan for the National Negro Health Movement, which the executive committee adopted. The plan, which drew on discussions from previous health week planning committee meetings, identified the need to increase the number of black doctors and nurses hired by government and voluntary organizations. It called for continuation of Negro Health Week observances, promotion of health education in black schools, and assistance to the health projects of voluntary organizations. It also recommended analysis of the 1930 U.S. census to determine black health status and access to health services.[33]

Much of the control at the national level over the direction of the Negro Health Week effort shifted in the late 1920s from those who had started it — laymen, mostly educators — to black doctors in the NMA. Educators led the movement at Tuskegee Institute in the 1910s and 1920s, then physicians at Howard University Medical School for a brief period from 1930 to 1932, until Brown took over at the Office of Negro Health Work.[34] By the late 1920s it was clear that Tuskegee Institute could no longer afford the administrative costs of coordinating National Negro Health Week. In 1929 plans were made to secure an underwriter to cover the expenses of running a national black health program and to pay the salary of someone to administer it.[35] Dr. Will W. Alexander, secretary of the NMA, wrote to Acting Surgeon General C. C. Pierce of the need for a black administrator:

> It seems to me highly desirable that there should be a Negro staff member of the Public Health Service who could work with the Department, first, in keeping Negro organizations working together on health education and, second, such a man could be of great value in keeping in close personal contact with the state departments of health, particularly in the South, and with other

health agencies that are trying to meet the special problems involved in Negro health conditions.

Alexander concluded with a reminder that efforts to improve black health would benefit the entire nation. "Of course," he noted, "I need not emphasize to you the special importance of Negro health in the general health program of the country."[36]

That same year, evidently unaware that this change was taking place, Dr. C. A. Lanon of Pennsylvania attacked Tuskegee leaders for not turning the health week effort over to the NMA. Lanon argued that it was an insult that the NMA had not been "invited or accredited a place of authority in the original scheme." Lanon concluded that "failure to consider the N.M.A. means failure of those earnestly desiring the hygienic and economic success of Negro Health Week."[37] Ironically, he raised this issue at the time that Robert Moton and Monroe Work were eager to turn over movement leadership to the NMA and the USPHS.

Black Health Education: The Office of Negro Health Work and the National Negro Health Movement

Brown owed his employment at the Office of Negro Health Work in the USPHS to his own diligence, financial support from a white philanthropic organization, and the intensive lobbying efforts of leaders at Tuskegee Institute and the NMA. Since at least 1917, leaders of the black medical association had wanted an "insider" to advocate federal health policy that was attentive to the needs of African Americans. They believed it was essential that the USPHS hire a black doctor.[38] As head of Tuskegee Institute, Moton insisted that someone must be appointed to the staff of the USPHS to carry out a year-round black health program, a position Brown desperately wanted and eventually received. In 1932 the USPHS rehired him to run the new Office of Negro Health Work (see Figure 2).[39]

When National Negro Health Week had its headquarters at Howard University, a black college in Washington, D.C., Brown was hired as the field secretary, or national organizer. His office was in the Department of Public Health at Howard University Medical School under the supervision of Dr. Algernon Jackson, the same man who in 1915 had queried Washington over the role of the NMA. Brown only received the job after urgent lobbying efforts. Facing dire financial troubles in 1930 as the Depression

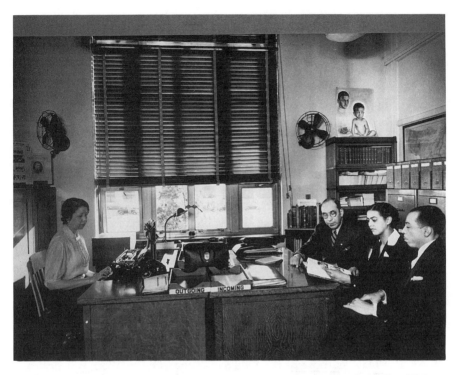

Figure 2. Dr. Roscoe C. Brown (center) with secretary and visitors in the Office of Negro Health Work, United States Public Health Service. Courtesy of the National Archives, Washington, D.C.

hit, he desperately wanted the job as field secretary. For ten years he had promoted National Negro Health Week, often without pay or with only minor reimbursement from the USPHS, and he argued that he had earned the position. "I must ask for the aid I deserve and now need," he explained to Moton. "I have been efficient, industrious and loyal in my work. It is asking too much to have me suffer loss and deprivation."[40]

The Julius Rosenwald Fund, a white philanthropic organization, provided the financial assistance needed to hire him. The organization donated $10,000 to cover part of Brown's salary as field secretary for several years.[41] About 10 percent (or one million dollars) of the fund's budget went to address black health issues from 1928 until financial allocations ended in 1942. Most of the money, over $800,000, went to the establishment and improvement of black hospitals, but the fund also provided some salary assistance to health departments to encourage them to hire black doctors.

The fund claimed credit for the employment of thirteen black doctors in state health departments across the country, including the South.[42] It also provided the money for the U.S. Children's Bureau, in the Department of Labor, to hire Dr. Walter Maddux in 1936 to provide education in obstetrics and pediatrics to southern black physicians.[43]

In 1932 Brown moved to the new Office of Negro Health Work, where he continued his activity as a paid organizer for National Negro Health Week and its year-round umbrella campaign, the National Negro Health Movement. He spent much of his time traveling around the country speaking to black organizations about health issues, holding workshops, and assisting community health campaigns. He was a dynamic, enthusiastic public lecturer, often in demand for health week lectures. In 1933, for example, he spent over one hundred days out in the field visiting forty-six communities in eight states, and in 1938 he traveled over 150 days to thirty communities in fifteen states.[44] He tried to raise the "health consciousness" of black Americans as well as promote interest in black health within white health agencies. He encouraged black Americans to take an active interest in their own health, stating: "Do not wait for the health department and other health agencies to seek you. The initiative should be exercised by the individual person, the home, and the neighborhood."[45]

The main purpose of the Office of Negro Health Work was health education. With a staff consisting only of Brown and a woman who worked as the secretary, the Office of Negro Health Work did not so much create health policy and black health projects as house the National Negro Health Movement and serve as an informational clearinghouse for the health activities of local communities. Brown produced radio broadcasts and health week sermons for National Negro Health Week. He provided voluntary organizations, health activists, and government agencies, such as state boards of health, with promotional materials for Negro Health Week, including posters, bulletins, and a newsletter. Finally, Brown was the editor of the newsletter *National Negro Health News*, a thick quarterly journal published from 1933 to 1950. This publication was a rich reservoir of information about black health concerns, including reports about health week activities and a range of black health topics, including information about hospitals, health professionals, health status, and health reform.

THE GROWTH OF THE NATIONAL NEGRO HEALTH MOVEMENT

National Negro Health Week and the year-round National Negro Health Movement together constituted a cross between an organization and a social movement. Like an organization, there was a headquarters, an executive committee and planning committee, and "turf battles" waged over control of national leadership. Like a social movement, the key activity took place in autonomous, community-led health campaigns that built on available resources wherever black people lived. Despite the attempt of black male leaders, especially doctors, to control the direction of the National Negro Health Movement, it remained a locally based grassroots movement. Even when the executive committee set priorities for the focus of annual health week campaigns, it had no power to enforce policy decisions upon local community organizers. For example, although Brown and his committees selected themes for Negro Health Week, such as the 1943 theme of "Health on the Home Front — Victory on the War Front," each community decided its specific health programs.[46]

Community campaigns focused on topics that were most relevant to the local circumstances. Brown identified three main components to community observances of Negro Health Week: (1) "clean-up work," such as painting, planting, and repairing homes and community buildings; (2) "educational work," such as health lectures, films, newspaper articles, and health literature; and (3) "practical work," such as health clinics, examinations, and inoculations. Throughout the 1930s and 1940s communities placed increasing emphasis on the "practical work," calling on health professionals, while continuing their commitment to sanitation efforts and health education programs.[47]

Brown kept detailed records of the number of communities observing Negro Health Week each year, records that documented the growth of the National Negro Health Movement. Apparently, the Depression of the 1930s did not slow interest in Negro Health Week programs — if anything, interest seemed to increase. Following the 1932 health week celebration, Brown wrote to Moton: "You will be pleased to know that the results of the last Health Week observance excelled those of prior years, though many difficulties beset most communities and groups during the year."[48] Brown found dramatic growth in the number of communities after 1930, perhaps because he stimulated interest through his numerous community visits or because more communities decided to submit health week reports. He also continued Tuskegee's practice of issuing health week awards to the best community reports, no doubt to encourage submissions.

Health week observations took place in every state where African Americans lived, from small rural counties in Mississippi to major metropolitan areas like Chicago. For six years during the 1930s, even the Civilian

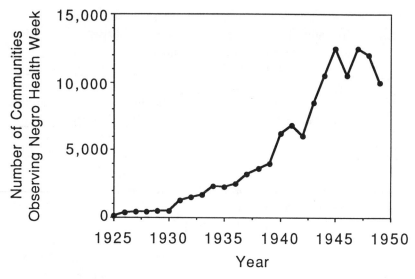

Figure 3. National Negro Health Week participation, 1925–1950.

Conservation Corps held Negro Health Week programs at its camps, and the National Youth Administration in Louisiana observed health week.[49] Negro Health Week campaigns appeared in places outside of the United States, including the Virgin Islands, a few African nations, and India, and during World War II Brown noted that "Health Week programs also were conducted among soldiers overseas," especially in England.[50]

The widespread community interest in Negro Health Week suggested that it was indeed a <u>mass movement</u>. Whereas in 1925 Tuskegee received notices of health week observances in 140 communities, in 1935 Brown received announcements from 2,200 communities at the Office of Negro Health Work. The piles of mail must have flooded his office. The number of health week reports, many of which included photographs of health week organizing committees and health week programs, peaked in 1945 when an astonishing 12,500 communities reported that they held Negro Health Week celebrations. Brown indicated that the number of people reached by National Negro Health Week activities dramatically increased from 500,000 in 1933 to five million in 1942 (see Figure 3).[51]

Ultimately, it was at the local level that people made this a grass-roots movement with possibilities for social transformation. The impressive growth of Negro Health Week participation demonstrates that African Americans, the professionals and the working poor, turned health week into a mass movement. The national executive committee made health policy and Brown spent weeks on the lecture circuit drumming up national interest, but people organizing in their own communities were the key to its success.

COMMUNITY ACTIVISM: NURSES, LAYWOMEN, AND PUBLIC HEALTH PRACTICE

The work of nurses and the voluntary public health labor of laywomen were essential to the creation of a mass movement. Nurses and laywomen addressed black needs at the community level and successfully mobilized community support for National Negro Health Week in urban areas and rural counties across the country. Much of women's community organizing involved the interaction of laywomen and public health nurses.

Throughout the early twentieth century the black nurse was a key figure in spreading the gospel of health to African Americans. As the field of public health nursing expanded in the twentieth century, and public health workers placed more emphasis on individual hygiene, nurses came to symbolize the ideal teachers. Public health nurses were especially important in rural areas where access to doctors was severely limited. Leaders of the black health movement agreed that "one of the greatest needs as related to public health work among Negroes is an adequate supply of well trained public health nurses."[52] Work believed that the public health nurse was "one of the most, if not the most," effective instructors in health education for black people.[53]

The number of public health nurses in the nation grew dramatically in the first half of the twentieth century. By the 1930s there were nearly 20,000 public health nurses. Public health nurses had more independence and autonomy than nurses in other fields. Public health nurses generally worked for voluntary agencies, like the American Red Cross, or government health departments. Many health departments hired nurses in the 1920s with funding from the Sheppard-Towner Act.[54]

Black nurses faced many difficulties in their struggle for professional recognition, their fight against segregation, and their efforts to meet the health needs of poor black people.[55] They faced discrimination in training, wages, and promotion. Yet by 1930 black nursing schools had produced some 5,000 black nurses.[56] By 1930 there were at least 470 black public health nurses in the country, 180 of whom worked in the South, where they constituted 20 percent of all public health nurses. By 1946 there were 1,100 black public health nurses in the United States. By the 1940s, when only 10 percent of all nurses were in public health work, 28 percent of black nurses found employment in public health.[57]

Black public health nurses actively recruited community women to assist in the task of health promotion in African-American communities. In 1929 in Virginia, financial assistance from the Rosenwald Fund enabled the state health department to hire Rosa Taylor, a black nurse. Because she was responsible for the health needs of black people in eight counties, an impossible task to perform alone, she organized health clubs to create connections with local women. Through the clubs she was able to reach many women at one time. The women of each club studied health education, met with the nurse every three months, and ran their own health projects, such as a program to immunize children against diphtheria.[58] From 1932 to 1937 nurses with the Virginia Department of Health organized similar health clubs for black mothers and midwives in thirty-two counties.[59]

Nurses, especially in rural areas, believed that working with women in their communities would encourage local interest in ongoing health work, as well as ease the nurses' burden. As Pearl McIver, a nursing director with the USPHS, noted:

> The efficient rural public health nurse realizes that the success of her program is largely dependent upon the interest and co-operation of the citizens of the community which she is serving. She knows that one is not greatly interested in a movement unless one has had a part in that movement and that assisting or participating in some small way is the surest way to create and to sustain interest in a program. She will make use of already organized clubs, lodges, or even ladies aid societies, getting these groups to form health committees, if such committees are not already in existence.[60]

Nurses and community women needed to work together because the task, especially in isolated rural areas, was so great.

Throughout the 1930s and 1940s black laywomen helped to create new health services and sustain existing ones in their communities, in part through contact with nurses. In southern Virginia, laywomen not only assisted the rural nurse with community health care but also defended the health department against the economic downturn of the Depression. One year the local black Mothers' Club assisted a woman whose husband had abandoned her and left her pregnant with no one to help. The midwife who delivered her had reported the case to a county nurse at the health department. The nurse gave the club leader a card that enabled her to get funds for the woman from the county poormaster, and six of the club women cleaned the woman's house and cooked her food. They also gave the woman a layette of baby clothes that the club women had made from sugar and flour sacks. Each day one of the club women came to the house to look after the mother and baby. According to McIver, "when the county health officials decided to do away with the health department a few months later, as an economy measure, these women and many others, made such a protest that the idea was soon abandoned and the health department was retained, in spite of the depression."[61]

The success of the black health movement, both in terms of obser-vances of Negro Health Week and the establishment of permanent health organizations, was due to the commitment of people at the grassroots level. Nurses played a vital role in promoting Negro Health Week programs and other black health projects, but they usually did not work alone.[62] For example, in 1940 Hyacinth Reid, a black nurse in Pennsylvania, served as chair of the health committee of the local branch of the National Associa-tion for the Advancement of Colored People (NAACP). She organized a Negro Health Week campaign with the assistance of young black women volunteers from the Pennsylvania Tuberculosis Society.[63]

Rural African Americans were as eager as urban residents to support public health work. Twenty-three residents of Saint Mary's County in Maryland assisted with their sixth observance of Negro Health Week, and according to the authors of the health week report,

> what we have accomplished has been done entirely through the country peo-ple themselves, working in cooperation with the Chairman and Secretary of this organization. There were no trained workers, other than these two. The work was done after school hours, at night, and on Sundays.[64]

The volunteers were both Protestants and Catholics, including six priests. Evidently this cooperation was a major accomplishment in itself; the health week report stated that "this seems worth mentioning in a territory where religious feeling has always been pronounced. One backward minister for-bade his congregation to participate, but they participated anyway." Ac-cording to the health week report, the county health officer was an alcoholic who failed to assist either the black or white citizens, so they had to create their own public health program.[65]

Public health organizers had little difficulty attracting audiences for health education programs despite white beliefs about apathy among rural black people and indifference to poor health conditions. In 1930 in Wicomico County, Maryland, the county ran health week by organizing every black school and providing children with health examinations. There were also public meetings with health lectures in five communities, and according to Dr. R. H. Riley, director of the Maryland health department, "the discussion went well into the night, showing that the negroes were interested and wanted to know what they could do to improve their health." Black community members established several permanent health committees to work on black health issues year-round, and they assisted the health department by providing transportation to health clinics as well as reporting the existence of contagious diseases. Nurses also conducted health education classes for black women, who in turn provided health information to their neighbors.[66]

Even the very poor took an active part in improving health conditions. Black tenant farmers in East Carroll Parish, a small delta county in Louisiana, also created a health week campaign. According to Dr. M. V. Hargett, director of the county health department, in 1930 Negro Health Week was "100 percent in the hands of the colored people and the accomplishments recorded represent what they did under their own leadership and initiative." Negro Health Week existed because of the joint efforts of the local health department, a public health nurse, and the local people. The health department sponsored the program, and a black nurse, Ala Mae Stephens, supervised the campaign and assisted in contacting churches, schools, and newspapers to promote health week. According to the health week report, organizers tried to instill an interest in "washing teeth, taking baths, cleaning homes, sunning beddings, killing bed bugs, repairing privies, cleaning up yards and papering houses." Furthermore, the people secured previously unavailable garbage removal services from a local town.[67]

Laywomen's community health work greatly increased the possibility that people would actually attend health clinics. In 1948 black women members of a health council in Montgomery County, Maryland, tried to improve black access to the services of their local health department. They assisted public health nurses at clinics and raised money to buy incubators for babies. They even purchased cars in order to drive rural patients to the health clinics.[68]

Black women's organizing efforts at the community level sustained a black health movement that targeted health improvement as a means to racial advancement. Although not a confrontational protest movement, the cumulative effect of health activism in thousands of rural and urban communities across the country was the creation of a mass movement that turned to the health arena to keep alive the black struggle for equality.

The Politics of Integration and the Black Health Movement

Black leaders after 1930 continued to argue that the attainment of equal rights depended first of all on the survival of the race. A 1944 editorial in the *Philadelphia Afro-American* reminded its readers that the end of World War II would not end the causes of ill-health, such as malnutrition and poor housing. Therefore black people had to continue to fight against the conditions that gave rise to poor health because "all our hopes for racial freedom and security in the post-war world are founded on the measure of our physical ability to survive."[69]

The more evidence that government health officials collected, the more that black health appeared to be a problem. By the 1930s statistical information on morbidity and mortality was available for every state for the first time, enabling public health officials to better determine the demographic breakdown of health problems, but also requiring them to explain the findings. Health department use of vital statistics increased the visibility of black health needs, but often led officials to blame the behavior of African Americans for their high rates of illness rather than investigating socioeconomic causes.

When urban centers and states with large black populations proved to have high morbidity rates, alarmed health officials justified the figures by blaming black communities. For example, in 1931 the USPHS made a survey of venereal disease in Baltimore and discovered very high rates, especially among the black population, that white health officials concluded was the result of black sexual immorality. The city responded with health campaigns, including observances of Negro Health Week, that stressed the dangers of unrestrained sexuality. Ten years later, when blood tests of enlistees for the military demonstrated that Baltimore had the second highest syphilis rate in the country, the health department again explained the situation by blaming the rate on the city's large black population.[70]

Throughout the 1930s and 1940s black leaders responded to such accusations by agreeing that the nation was only as healthy as its sickest members. "It is our belief that the country's health can be no better proportionately than that of the most neglected health segment of its population," proclaimed Walter White in 1947 when he contacted President Harry S

Truman on behalf of the NAACP.[71] Black leaders reminded local governments that high rates of disease could be addressed with preventive measures once racist practices ended and health departments provided services to all members of the community.[72] Increasingly, many black leaders saw "integration" as the only solution.

 By World War II some national black leaders argued for the end of annual black health week campaigns and in favor of the integration of African Americans into all aspects of the health care sector. Like their white counterparts, men like Dr. Montague Cobb of the NMA and Walter White of the NAACP were inclined to support a medical vision of health care and had little patience for the "outdated" methods of the National Negro Health Movement. They envisioned nurses and doctors, hospitals, and medical technology as the weapons in the fight against disease, not community clean-up campaigns and health education programs by layworkers.

The struggle to integrate hospitals, medical and nursing schools, and medical and nursing associations became known as the medical civil rights movement.[73] The movement directly confronted segregation itself, not just inequality within a segregated system. In 1947 White summed up his philosophy for racial advancement when he stated that Negroes deserved to share "identically" with other citizens in all medical institutions and health programs.[74]

The resistance to hospital segregation came from black community people as well as leaders because of numerous life-threatening encounters with "white-only" policies. For example, Pearl Miles of Washington, D.C. lodged a formal complaint when a white hospital denied her sister admission when she was in labor. At 5:00 A.M. on December 22, 1944, Pearl Miles watched her sister give birth on a sidewalk in Washington, D.C., within half a block of the Sibley Hospital because it had a white-only policy and refused to admit the black woman. The women had been walking to Gallinger Hospital, which accepted black patients, when the pregnant woman collapsed on the sidewalk just outside Sibley Hospital. Pearl Miles ran into Sibley Hospital to get assistance and encountered a white nurse who refused to summon a doctor and only reluctantly agreed to offer first aid in the basement. Insulted and rejected by the hospital, the sisters waited outside in subfreezing weather for twenty minutes until an ambulance came and took them to Gallinger Hospital.[75] Later Pearl Miles filed an affidavit with the National Council of Negro Women, an umbrella organization of black women's groups with headquarters in Washington, D.C.[76] Like so many other cases, there is no indication that her sister received any compensation.

Well after 1950 the black dream of access to white health institutions remained a dream deferred. As Dr. Paul B. Cornely of Howard University Medical School pointed out, access to scientific medicine came slowly to black America in general, and black rural Southerners in particular, because of the extreme shortage of medical personnel and facilities as well as white resistance to integration. Until such time as medical facilities and personnel were available, everyone who had some skills contributed to black health, even in the post-World War II era.[77]

To Brown, integrating white medical institutions was an admirable but long-term goal, meaningful only to the middle class. As black calls for integration in the post-World War II era gained ascendancy, Brown continued to believe that black Americans, especially the poor, needed separate black services. He described his work and that of others in the National Negro Health Movement as providing assistance from "those who know and serve" to "those who need and seek."[78] He thought that lofty visions were fine but he was realistic and knew black communities still had immediate survival needs that had to be addressed. In 1949 he acknowledged the positive legal efforts to force integration, but still maintained that "while State and Federal legislation may be necessary to give the Negro a better chance to enjoy good health and long life, the National Negro Health Week and other voluntary movements offer immediate programs through which the Negro and his community can secure some improvement in present conditions."[79]

Contemporary critics charged Brown with taking a retrogressive "accommodationist" stance, as opposed to the progressive position of "integrationists." In the post-World War II era, many black activists steadfastly believed that segregation was on the way out and complete equality was the only acceptable option. In this view, men like Brown stood in the way by strengthening segregation in their willingness to strike a bargain and settle for separate services as long as black people had access to something. The debate over political strategy for black health improvement raged on, building on the positions once associated with Booker T. Washington and W. E. B. Du Bois. In much the same way the differences were outweighed by the shared commitment to racial equality and improved health.

"No Such Thing as Negro Health": The End of an Era

In 1950 the USPHS pronounced the end of the National Negro Health Movement and the Office of Negro Health Work on the grounds that the nation was moving toward integration. According to Brown, a government evaluation of the Office of Negro Health Work had determined there was "the need for integration" of the work previously performed separately for black health by the office.[80] In announcing the termination of the black health program at the USPHS, Federal Security Administrator Oscar R. Ewing stated that it was "in keeping with the trend toward integration of all programs for the advancement of the people in the fundamentals of health education and welfare."[81]

Brown's own thoughts on the demise of the black health program and the justification put forth by the government are difficult to decipher from his official reports. In the final issue of *National Negro Health News* in 1950, Brown wrote:

> Eighteen years ago there was a pressing need to focus attention on the particular health problems of the Negro and to concentrate efforts in a national Negro health movement. Today, we know that this movement has been successful . . . so successful that there is not the same urgency to emphasize separate needs. Rather the trend now is for all groups to work together for mutual welfare.[82]

It may have been difficult for him to witness the end of an era in which he had invested so much of his life, but he tried to portray it in a positive light.

Black health activism at the community level and, to a lesser degree, within the federal government did make a difference during the first half of the twentieth century. Brown concluded that "the health of the Negro and his community has improved through the years of the National Negro Health Week movement."[83] In the last issue of the *National Negro Health News* he pointed to statistics that indicated black morbidity and mortality rates had dropped significantly over the decades, despite the fact that they were consistently higher than white rates. Black infant mortality rates, for example, declined from 180 per 1,000 live births in 1915 to 48 per 1,000 in 1947. Yet Brown reminded his readers that the black infant mortality rate was still 60 percent higher than the white rate. Life expectancy had increased for black Americans, from about 34 years for men and 38 for women in 1910 to about 58 years for men and 62 years for women in 1947. Yet despite such gains, on average African Americans did not live as long as whites.[84]

Although black health activities at the grassroots level no doubt continued even after the formal administration of the National Negro Health Movement ended, 1950 did mark a turning point. Concerned about the future of public health work for African Americans, Brown recommended

that local communities take inventory of Negro Health Week accomplishments in their areas and evaluate future needs. He advised community
health week supporters to

> determine what next steps to take to maintain the benefits derived from the
> Health Week activities and to use more largely and effectively the health re-
> sources available to them in their own communities — their family doctors,
> health departments and voluntary health agencies, and the community in-
> stitutions and organizations related to health education, conservation, and
> promotion.[85]

He wanted the struggle to continue, even if he was no longer able to help
organize it.

With the end of the health campaign, Brown was transfered to a new
branch in the USPHS. U.S. Surgeon General Leonard Scheele, who replaced Thomas Parran in 1948, appointed Brown head of a new Special
Programs Branch of the Division of Health Education. The position, undoubtedly a concession to Brown who was approaching retirement anyway,
required him to address all minority health concerns, which allowed Brown
to continue to provide consultation to black community organizations.[86]
Brown retired in 1954 at age seventy after a distinguished career in public
health.[87] Before his death in 1962, Brown received many honors from his
peers, including awards from Howard University, the USPHS, and the
American Public Health Association.

For Brown, it was a sad ending to a long career, but several other black
leaders were delighted to see the end of a health campaign that they saw as
a symbol of segregation. Dr. Montague Cobb, who taught at Howard
University, stated that "the idea of a special 'Negro Health Week' has become outmoded."[88] In an article in the *Journal of the National Medical Association*, Cobb announced the termination of the *National Negro Health
News*, noting:

> now that it is accepted generally that "health is everybody's business," the need
> for such a publication is no longer apparent. The Journal congratulates Health
> News for its valuable service and the Public Health Service for its foresight in
> establishing an integrated program of survey and activity schedule.[89]

Cobb and his black medical organization in Washington, D.C., the Medico-
Chirurgical Society, believed that separate health programs and facilities
"no matter how good do not compensate for failure of integration. The
ghetto no matter how beautiful is still a ghetto."[90]

Dr. Louis T. Wright, who was a leader of the NAACP along with Cobb and White, had publicly opposed National Negro Health Week as early as 1938. Wright, a 1915 graduate of Harvard Medical School, made his reputation at Harlem Hospital in New York.[91] Wright helped organize the Manhattan Medical Society in 1930, breaking away from the original black medical society in New York over political philosophy. He and some other doctors had wanted full integration in hospitals and criticized the Rosenwald Fund for supporting separate black hospitals, which other black New York doctors saw as beneficial.[92] In 1938 Wright spoke out directly against Negro Health Week in a newspaper interview, stating that black Americans deserved the same year-round health programs as white Americans and that the Manhattan Medical Society refused to observe Negro Health Week. According to the newspaper article, entitled "Dr. Wright Socks Health Week in the Eye," Wright remarked: "Why should we be singled out for a health week celebration any more than any other group?"[93]

Leaders such as Wright and Cobb argued that separate health programs should never be endorsed, no matter what the short-term loss to individuals, because they supported the notion of black inferiority. In 1938 Wright and T. Arnold Hill of the National Urban League had presented a joint statement at a National Health Conference in Washington, D.C., opposing the second-class status of black Americans. They stated: "There is no such thing as Negro health. Disease draws no color line, but one would never know this from the way in which health services are administered in most places in this country." Their position was that there could be "no compromise with segregation if the Negro's health is to be permanently bettered."[94] In 1952 Wright repeated this position when he suggested that separate black programs should not be accepted even for humanitarian reasons. "This is a case where the greater good was served by denying to some of our group the immediate benefit of a segregated set-up, and it represents a casualty in this all-out war against discrimination and segregation," he explained.[95]

Conclusion

The mid-twentieth century was an era of transition as the black health movement's political strategy gave way to demands for integration. National leaders like Brown were on their way out, to be replaced by men like Cobb. Some doctors, like Cornely of the Department of Public Health at

Howard University Medical School and past president of the American Public Health Association, straddled the eras of segregation and of integration, playing an active role in each.

Cornely, who would help lead the medical civil rights movement, nevertheless believed that programs such as National Negro Health Week provided important benefits. He believed that the black health movement played a vital role, especially among the poor in southern rural communities. Cornely, who had been active in the National Negro Health Movement since the 1930s, occasionally spoke at Negro Health Week celebrations. Aware of the criticisms of the movement, he still believed that it had been a catalyst for advancing black rights. When interviewed in the late 1980s, he recalled that even though the movement did not have confrontational moments like current civil rights struggles, it did open some doors for African Americans.[96]

Due to the limited financial and personnel support from the federal government, the National Negro Health Movement had great but unrealized potential to save lives. Despite over thirty years of service with the USPHS, Brown was never able to carry out many of his plans. Indeed, it appears that the USPHS never paid serious attention to Brown and the Office of Negro Health Work. Cornely suggested that the USPHS merely tried to appease African Americans with an underfunded, understaffed program instead of any serious commitment to improving black health. In his view, the USPHS marginalized the Office of Negro Health Work and isolated it from the rest of the health departments. Cobb concurred that the USPHS had merely tolerated Brown and his work. The white public health establishment never even properly rewarded Brown for his years of service as a government public health official when, to Brown's great disappointment, the USPHS failed to make him a commissioned officer. As was standard practice before 1947, the USPHS classified him as a Negro specialist with no rank.[97]

Black health leaders had hoped to shape federal health and welfare policy through appointments of black personnel, believing that they would best represent black interests in the development and administration of government policy. Brown's experience at the USPHS illustrates the difficulties encountered by black government officials, whose work was repeatedly circumscribed. Yet, Brown's very presence within the USPHS was a sign of change. As his career demonstrated, President Franklin Roosevelt's "Black Cabinet" was as much a concession to black demands as a sign of Roosevelt's liberalism. Having black advisors was a significant departure from previous administrations, but one that African Americans had a hand in creating.[98]

Ultimately, the federal government failed African Americans and they had to construct their own health policy and practice to meet the needs of black America. At the local level, black community health activism during the 1930s and 1940s, often led by black women, provided a measure of health provisions to communities generally neglected by the white health establishments. The black middle class and the working poor, health professionals and layworkers alike, constructed the National Negro Health Movement out of a shared commitment to survival. In the words of one of the local black health organizers, black public health work "awakened in the Negro awareness of his condition and his power to do something about these problems." It also demonstrated to white people "that Negroes can organize and carry through programs of welfare for and among themselves."[99]

In the final analysis, the federal government and New Deal programs did not save black America—African Americans rescued themselves. Furthermore, as the next chapter shows, government interest in black health was not without its price. Ironically, federal attention to disease in black Americans could have a detrimental impact on the health of the black poor.

Part II

The Implementation of
Black Health Programs

4. Good Intentions and Bad Blood in Alabama

From the Tuskegee Movable School to the Tuskegee Syphilis Experiment

Throughout the history of the black health movement, black reformers tried to secure social services for the rural poor by turning to the federal government to circumvent the inequality of the Jim Crow South. They viewed the acquisition of federal assistance as a political victory because it was a way to bypass the restrictions of local white-only policies and states' rights justifications for systematically denying social welfare funds to African Americans. Yet, as the histories of the Tuskegee Movable School and the Tuskegee Syphilis Study illustrate, government involvement proved to have oppressive as well as progressive consequences for poor African Americans.

Black professionals risked little by linking their social welfare programs to federal initiatives, as long as they maintained control over their own agenda. For example, Booker T. Washington convinced the federal government to incorporate the Tuskegee Movable School, a black rural development program he directed, within the extension service work funded by the U.S. Department of Agriculture. This action set a precedent for federal government support to black farmworkers and marked the beginning of organized black agricultural extension work in the United States. From 1906 to 1944 the Tuskegee Movable School provided adult education programs in agriculture, home economics, and health for rural African Americans throughout Alabama. This traveling school became a model for the creation of rural development programs in other states, such as Mississippi, and even other countries, such as India.[1]

Black professionals counted on the benefits of government involvement to outweigh the costs to the poor. In the case of the Tuskegee Movable School they were undoubtedly right, but as the history of the Tuskegee Syphilis Study shows, there were dire consequences when they were wrong. From 1932 to 1972 white physicians of the United States Public Health

Service (USPHS) carried out a "study" on approximately 400 rural black men in Macon County, Alabama. The study, which historian James Jones has described as "the longest nontherapeutic experiment on human beings in medical history," was predicated on following the course of untreated syphilis until death.[2]

Black health workers and educators at Tuskegee Institute played a critical role in the government's syphilis experiment. Robert Moton, head of Tuskegee Institute, and Dr. Eugene Dibble, the medical director of Tuskegee's hospital, both lent their endorsement and institutional resources to the government study. However, no one was more vital to the experiment than Eunice Rivers (Laurie), a black public health nurse. Rivers worked in the public health field from 1923 until well after her retirement in 1965. She began her career with the Tuskegee Institute Movable School during the 1920s, and after a decade of service she became involved in the infamous Tuskegee Syphilis Study. In her capacity as a public health nurse, Rivers acted as the liaison between the men in the study and the doctors of the USPHS. Indeed, Rivers was the key to maintaining subject interest in the experiment for forty years.[3] Paradoxically, it is a "tribute" to her years of hard work at developing relationships with people in the surrounding countryside through her public health work with the Tuskegee Movable School that the men in the Tuskegee Syphilis Study continued to cooperate year after year.

How could black professionals, including health workers dedicated to preserving life, participate in such a project? Historians have focused on the study as scientifically unjustifiable and as an unethical experiment that highlighted the racism of American medicine and the federal government. While affirming the validity of these assessments, I return to the troubling question of the role of Tuskegee Institute's black professionals. This chapter demonstrates that their participation can best be understood when set within the context of twentieth-century public health work. The histories of the Tuskegee Movable School and the Tuskegee Syphilis Study raise important questions about the gendered nature of public health work, the constraints on black middle-class reform efforts, and the costs and benefits to the poor.

Rural African Americans and the Tuskegee Community

The Tuskegee Movable School was unique among rural development programs by and for African Americans in that it drew on the extensive human resources and political connections of Tuskegee Institute, located in Macon County, Alabama. As we have seen, Tuskegee Institute served as headquarters for numerous reform efforts by black professionals who wanted to bring their vision of the benefits of the twentieth century to those at the bottom of the socioeconomic ladder. Black educators, social workers, and health workers tried to bring enlightenment and a better standard of living to the rural black poor through the improvement of crops, houses, health, education, and morals. Washington relied on a solid network of black educators and former students to garner support for his various campaigns, and together with lucrative connections to wealthy white businessmen and government officials, Washington and his assistants carried out a number of programs for rural black Southerners. The Annual Tuskegee Negro Conference, National Negro Health Week, and the Tuskegee Movable School are examples of Tuskegee's racial uplift work for people in the surrounding countryside.[4]

In the spirit of Tuskegee Institute's educational philosophy, black extension agents from the Tuskegee Movable School tried to turn black tenant farmers into healthy, thrifty landowners. Although it is difficult to uncover the voices of rural African Americans who participated in extension service programs, and much of the following draws on the reports of a few extension service leaders, general patterns of interactions between the "students" and the instructors are discernable.

In their government reports, black extension workers sometimes appeared to deny the importance of deeper structural barriers, and they implied that black tenants could all be landowners if they just altered their behavior. It is difficult to know if such sentiments represented their assessments of the rural poor or their strategies with the white establishment, given that much of what we know about the work of the extension agents comes from statistical and narrative reports submitted to government officials. Agents no doubt censored themselves in an effort to tell officials what they wanted to hear and what would most likely benefit black programs.

Poor rural African Americans shared the vision that landownership was a key to black freedom from white control. They wanted to become independent landowners and homeowners instead of sharecroppers and tenant farmers working for white planters. Landownership among black Southerners actually increased between 1880 and World War I. By 1910, of the 850,000 African Americans who farmed land in the South, nearly 200,000 were landowners. However, most farms owned by African Americans in the early twentieth century were small and on poor soil. Furthermore, as the history of lynching demonstrates, African Americans faced the danger of white retaliation for black economic success. It was not uncommon for white people to find legal and extralegal methods to force black people to lose their land or sell it at a loss.[5]

Although most African Americans lived in the rural South working in agriculture until well into the Great Depression, they were usually not landowners. For example, in Alabama as in other Deep South states, most African Americans worked on white-owned cotton plantations as tenant farmers. In 1925, 90 percent of the rural African Americans in Macon County were tenant farmers, while almost half of the white people in the county were landowners. As tenants, black people rented land from a landlord and paid rent either in cash or in a share (usually half) of the crop, known as sharecropping. Black sharecroppers were even more vulnerable to white exploitation than black landowners. For example, black tenants often paid higher rent and interest rates than white tenants. All these factors contributed to a situation in which many rural African Americans were trapped in a cycle of debt and poverty.[6]

In the early twentieth century, most rural African Americans lived in unhealthy surroundings with few modern amenities. They faced a range of health problems including malaria, typhoid fever, hookworm disease, pellagra, and venereal disease, along with malnutrition and high infant and maternal mortality rates. One black extension service agent for the Tuskegee Movable School, Thomas Monroe Campbell, wrote that in his work he encountered

> hundreds of squalid, ramshackled cabins, tenanted by forlorn, emaciated, poverty stricken Negroes who year after year struggled in cotton fields and disease-laden swamps, trying to eke out a miserable existence.[7]

Homes had few screens, window panes, or even windows, and few sanitary toilets. T. J. Woofter of the Commission on Interracial Cooperation reported that "it has been said of some of the houses that the school children can return home and study geology through the floor, botany through the sides, and astronomy through the roof."[8] In terms of material conditions, most rural African Americans barely had the essentials.

Black and White Extension Service Work

The federal government funded southern extension service work in order to improve agricultural production, create a contented labor force, and reduce migration out of rural areas.[9] Black and white extension agents struggled to fight the boll weevil, a beetle that destroyed cotton crops in every county in Alabama by 1916. However, black extension service work differed from white programs. White agricultural extension agents usually geared their crop improvement work toward helping landowners and promoted cash crops and commercial farming. Meanwhile, black agents focused on subsistence farming and the development of economic independence.[10]

There were far fewer black extension agents than white agents, despite the large number of black agricultural workers in the South. For example, in the 1910s across the nation there were only a few black agents; by World War I there were two hundred; and by the 1930s not quite four hundred black male and female agents. Many of these agents were graduates of Tuskegee Institute, Hampton Institute, and Florida Agricultural and Mechanical College.[11]

The salaries of extension service agents varied by both race and gender. For example, by World War I white male agents received about $135 per month compared to $75 for black men. White women received about $75 per month, much less than their male counterparts, but still more than the usual $60 received by black women. One state extension director admitted that when it came to salary, "we allowed these agents just as little as we thought they could possibly get along with," leading some white female agents in Alabama to complain that "the expense of doing the work was greater than the salary."[12]

The work of black and white extension service agents differed in some respects but it shared a gendered division of labor. While male farm agents focused on educating men about agriculture, female home demonstration agents focused on educating women about home economics and family care. Although some of the activities of the male extension agents had important health ramifications, most health work fell within the women's domain. In isolated rural areas, home demonstration agents and nurses disseminated vital health information about hygiene and sanitation to poor women who carried the burden of health care provisions.

A Farmer's College on Wheels: The Tuskegee Movable School

Washington referred to the Tuskegee Movable School as "A Farmer's College on Wheels." The first Movable School was a mule-drawn wagon built by students at Tuskegee Institute in 1906. It carried equipment and personnel, and it was known as the Jesup Agricultural Wagon in honor of the New

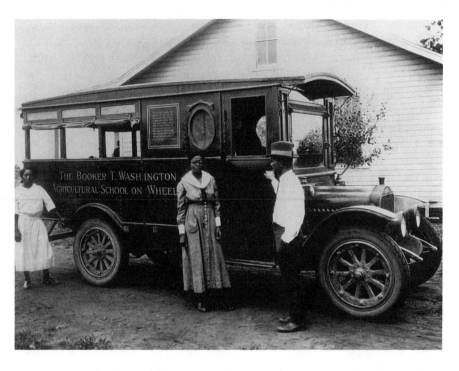

Figure 4. From left to right: Home demonstration agent Luella C. Hanna, public health nurse Eunice Rivers, and unidentified farm agent, rural workers for the Tuskegee Institute Movable School, Alabama, 1923. Courtesy of the National Archives, Washington, D.C.

York banker Morris K. Jesup, who assisted with the expenses of building it. Washington also garnered endorsement and financial support from John D. Rockefeller's General Education Board.[13] In 1918 Tuskegee replaced the old cart and mules for an automobile called the Knapp Agricultural Truck, named after Seaman Knapp, who created farm demonstration work. This truck eased transportation difficulties tremendously while providing more space for equipment and personnel. Then in 1923, after it broke down, 30,000 black farmers and a few white people donated $5,000 to buy a new truck, which was called the Booker T. Washington Agricultural School on Wheels. Each of these vehicles served at one time as the Tuskegee Movable School (see Figure 4).[14]

   Although the Tuskegee Movable School was initially set up by men for men, the personnel expanded over the years to include women. From 1906 until 1915 the school had only a few male farm agents, then in 1915 the school added a female home demonstration agent, and in 1920 the school added a public health nurse to the crew. Usually a total of three or four agents traveled together with the school.

THE FARM AGENT IN THE FIELD

The black male farm agent of the Movable School was in charge of addressing agricultural problems. Throughout the 1910s and 1920s black farm agents, whether with the Movable School or in other black extension service programs in the South, taught crop diversification (growing crops other than just cotton) as a way to limit the damage to agricultural production done by the boll weevil.[15] Agents taught how to use modern farm equipment, terrace land, prune fruit trees, raise pigs, build steps, measure and cut lumber, mix concrete, and make whitewash to use on houses and fences. Many of the projects had ramifications for the improvement of health, especially putting screens on windows to guard against flies and mosquitoes and installing sanitary toilets to prevent disease.[16]

Thomas Monroe Campbell (1883–1956), hired to work for the Movable School in 1906, became the first black farm agent of the U.S. Department of Agriculture and later the head of black extension work in the lower South. Campbell, who was born in Georgia on a white-owned farm, believed his own rural background assisted him in reaching poor black tenant farmers. When Campbell was about five years old, his mother convinced his father, who was a tenant farmer and Methodist preacher, to buy a small tract of land outside of town. Not long after, his mother died, leaving six children and a large doctor's bill. In order to pay the bill his father mortgaged the home and the land, and eventually lost both. Campbell remembered that "from that time on I worked with my father on various plantations until I was 15 years old, and then I decided definitely to get an education at any cost."[17] Campbell eventually attended Tuskegee Institute and graduated in 1906 with a diploma in agriculture. He assisted with the annual farmers' conferences and drove the carriage for Washington. After his graduation Washington hired him as a farm agent and then as head of the Movable School.

THE HOME DEMONSTRATION AGENT: PROMOTING GOOD HOUSEKEEPING

The lessons of the home demonstration agent in home economics were as essential to rural development and the work of the Movable School as that of farm agents' sessions on agriculture. In several respects home demonstration agents were to rural women what settlement house workers were to urban immigrant women, agents of modernization and advocates for the poor.[18] Despite women's work in the fields, extension programs for women focused exclusively on improving women's work in the home. Sociologist Monroe Work expressed the idealized role for women in 1910 when he wrote that

> the women are spending the greater portion of their time, not in working in the fields, but in attending to household duties. They are making their homes neat and comfortable. They have a place and a special time to eat. The food is properly prepared, placed upon a table, and served in suitable dishes.[19]

Home demonstration agents taught rural women how to increase food production and preservation. Canning programs and canning clubs were very popular among both black and white women, especially as part of the war effort during World War I.[20]

The Movable School hired its first home demonstration agent, N. Juanita Coleman, in 1915 with funding through the federal Smith-Lever Act. Coleman had entered Tuskegee Institute in 1904 after earning the entrance fee and railroad fare by running a kindergarten in her home state of Texas. She graduated in 1908, and Margaret Murray Washington subsequently sent her to teach school at the nearby Elizabeth Russell Settlement. After teaching there a while, Coleman moved to Texas, where she taught school for several years. Then she worked as a home demonstration agent with the Movable School for six years until she became Margaret Washington's secretary in the early 1920s. Finally, in 1923 Coleman opened a hospital in Demopolis, Alabama, which she operated with money raised from donations.[21]

Home demonstration agents during the 1910s and 1920s attempted to train women in proper housekeeping techniques. They provided lessons in the best way to cook, clean, sew, and make soap, handicrafts, and cotton mattresses for sale and personal use. They provided instructions in how to repair clothing and bed linen, make curtains and rugs, do laundry, and raise poultry. Sometimes agents ran an electric line from the Movable School into the house to demonstrate such appliances as a washing machine, cream separator, butter churn, and electric iron, technology completely out of the financial reach of most rural women.[22]

In addition to housekeeping, female extension workers focused on family care and, in the process, shaped the health component of rural development work. Home demonstration agents brought health education, especially information on nutrition, sanitation, and hygiene, directly to rural women. They promoted observances of National Negro Health Week, assisted with baby clinics, and provided information on birth control and personal hygiene, such as bathing, washing one's hair, and brushing one's teeth. From World War I to World War II home demonstration agents emphasized clean homes, clean bodies, appropriate food and clothing, and good health.[23]

Black professionals, including extension workers, did not question women's primary responsibility for family health and therefore directed the vast majority of their health programs toward women. The training started early with the 4-H agricultural movement — hand, head, heart, and health — in which extension agents taught boys to think as future farmers and girls as future homemakers who would one day be in charge of the health of their families.

The underlying philosophy of home demonstration work was that, even if poor rural women could not buy modern conveniences, they could still enjoy the appearance of modern consumer culture. Indeed, by twentieth-century urban standards these were the bare necessities. For example, the home demonstration agent was supposed to assist rural women who had little or no financial resources to make home furnishings. According to extension worker accounts, the home demonstration agent helped women use available materials like wooden crates to create many useful items, such as clothes closets, dressing tables, and wash stands. Even a kitchen sink with plumbing was not beyond reach. Through garden and poultry sales women were able to remodel their kitchens and "install simple water systems" that had "a barrel on the outside of the house with faucet and sink on the inside." After filling the barrel with fresh water each morning, the family had indoor plumbing.[24]

No doubt rural black women, like poor women in general, made a little go a long way well before lessons from extension agents. Many rural homes had "a little make-believe porch, wooden blinds for windows, [and] a block of wood or an old bucket turned upside down for steps," according Movable School home demonstration agent Laura Daly. Daly, who replaced Coleman in the 1920s, learned that most of the women had managed to cover exposed rafters and walls in their homes with newspapers, magazine covers, and circus posters. Pages from the Sears catalogue proved useful for blocking holes in the wall as well as for toilet paper. Daly saw women use lard buckets "to cook in, milk in, wash dishes in, and bathe in." Many women had to do their family's laundry down at the spring. Daly noted that

> usually there is an attempt at a flower yard, but it and the [vegetable] garden if there is one, have a hard struggle for existence during the work season, for there is no time to attend to either of them, the chickens or the children save Saturday afternoon.[25]

Rural women were constantly busy with some task, whether working in the cotton fields; tending to the gardens, chickens, and children; or cooking, cleaning, and nursing the sick. Daly reported that rural people had little leisure time or entertainment opportunities, although she observed that some homes had a phonograph, piano, or organ, even if in poor condition.[26]

One of the major concerns of the home demonstration agent was to teach nutrition and improve the rural diet, which featured "just one fried meal after another," according to Daly.[27] Luella C. Hanna, Alabama state home demonstration agent for black women, explained that "the busy farm women must prepare three meals a day and must prepare them in the quickest possible way — which is to fry breakfast, fry dinner, and fry supper." Rural people who lived and worked on plantations often ate mainly pork meat, corn bread, and molasses because these items were inexpensive and could be purchased at the plantation store.[28]

Home demonstration agents knew that despite dominant gender prescriptions, women did agricultural labor on top of household labor, so sometimes agents geared their educational programs toward helping women cope with their double burden. As one solution, agents encouraged women to serve their families at least one boiled meal each day. They taught them how to construct a fireless cooker, or slow cooker, out of a wooden lard tub, using shredded corn shucks as a liner for insulation, a kettle for holding the food, a zinc bucket in which to place the kettle, and a two-inch-thick flat rock placed in the bottom of the bucket. Women were shown how to prepare a balanced meal in the fireless cooker while they were out working in the fields.[29]

In families with some financial resources, rural women tried to negotiate with their husbands for farm and home improvements by invoking the authority of extension service agents. Campbell saw evidence to suggest that women were the ones who convinced their men to carry out the changes recommended by agents, such as repairing steps, whitewashing the house, and improving the outhouse. At least one woman, who like many cooked in iron pots and frying pans over the fire hearth, was able to purchase a stove.[30] Daly recalled:

> I like to think of how happy one woman was over her first stove. She had put off having the home demonstration club meeting at her house because she cooked on the fireplace. Finally the next meeting was appointed for her home. The husband, embarrassed, brought his wife to town on the Saturday previous to the meeting day and purchased their first stove. They had been married more than fifteen years.[31]

The resources of many families were so limited that even purchasing on credit was an impossibility, but there were some women who used extension work to achieve these victories.

Home demonstration agents did on occasion act as advocates for rural women's self-development. For example, Daly believed that women's heavy work burden was responsible for their poor health. She saw women working from early in the morning until late at night providing care for their families and labor in the fields. During National Negro Health Week one year, she tried to focus attention specifically on women's health issues, "to make the farm woman more conscious of her duty towards keeping herself well, especially emphasizing what she herself could do in that direction." Daly said the problem was that "mothers and wives are given to thinking only in terms of comfort and consideration for their husbands and children."[32] For this reason, women agents occasionally offered a critique of women's position within families.

Rural Education on the Road and the Plantation

The educational philosophy of the Tuskegee Movable School, like that of all agricultural extension work, was to teach by example to a mostly illiterate clientele. As Thomas Campbell, one of the most prolific writers on black extension work, explained: "We realized that many farmers could not read or write, and for that reason we adhered to methods that they could see and hear and understand."[33] Extension agents believed they were most successful at changing people's behavior when they were able to develop personal relationships with them. Campbell reported that:

> The workers get into the lives of the farmers, and their families, first of all, by gaining their confidence. They converse with them in their own language about their problems, real and imaginary; they encourage parents to send

their children to school; they often spend nights around the fireside with them and listen to interesting stories pertaining to the local history of their communities.[34]

Agents were not supposed to just hand out literature or to lecture. They were supposed to become involved in the life of rural communities and then involve the people in educational demonstrations.

In order to keep attendance high, the agents tried not to hold sessions during the planting and harvesting seasons. They held most sessions during the winter break, from December to February, before people planted their crops and during the summer break, from July to September, before people gathered their crops. In this way the Movable School reached hundreds of people in Alabama. For example, in 1915 the school traveled for six weeks in eight counties and made contacts with 5,000 African Americans. In 1922 the Movable School reached 1,885 people in four counties in only a few weeks. In 1928 the school held sessions in fifty-four communities and reached 4,600 people.[35]

Selecting School Sites

Initially the extension workers held teaching sessions in black community institutions such as churches, schools, and courthouses, but by 1920 they decided they would reach more people by going directly to their homes. According to Coleman, the agents learned that they had to go directly to the plantations and farms if they wanted to reach the poorest class of farmers, the sharecroppers and tenants. As Coleman explained:

> We noticed that the class of people who needed these instructions most, were not attending these meetings and we were not coming in contact with them, because this class went to church only when there was preaching; rarely went to the schoolhouse because in too many cases they didn't like the teacher and the last time they were at the courthouse they felt that they had not been given a fair chance or justice.[36]

Coleman found that attendance increased and she could demonstrate her lessons more easily when agents went to people's homes.

Agents usually selected one of the poorer homes for their extension service demonstrations, concluding that a tenant farmer could not match the farm and home improvements made by a landowning neighbor. Agents were supposed to select the homes of residents who were on good terms with the rest of the community in order to ensure that people would come to the demonstrations and to allay any feelings of favoritism regarding the selection of one home over another.[37] Because the tenants had little or no resources, the landowner was supposed to pay for the necessary materials in exchange for free labor from people in the community who carried out the various farm and home improvement lessons.

Black extension agents often encountered plantation owners who resisted participating in programs that might alter their present arrangement with tenants. They feared that rural extension work would "disturb the established plantation relationships." Campbell and others discovered that "most plantation owners were pretty well satisfied with the existent tenant system and therefore were not so enthusiastic in encouraging Negroes to try new methods of farming."[38] Yet black agents had to find ways to work with the white planters, who expected them to exhibit proper deference, in order to help black tenant farmers and to keep their own jobs.

Black agents did manage to obtain approval from some white landowners for black extension work once they convinced them that the educational programs and improvements would help to secure a stable labor force and "make the tenants more contented and appreciative of their surroundings." Sometimes white planters even appeared at sessions to offer "words of encouragement."[39] In 1922 C. A. Patillo, a white plantation owner with a large number of black tenants, urged his renters to attend the Movable School and agreed to pay for the cost of materials. He wrote to the white county agent that he thought the project would help tenants to "realize that they can make a great deal more net profit by improving their methods."[40] Clearly, it was easier for him to blame the poverty of tenant farmers on their "methods" rather than the labor system from which he benefited.

CONVINCING CLIENTS TO COME

One of the ways that agents convinced local people to participate in the Movable School, in addition to whatever pressure plantation owners brought to bear, was through contacting local black community leaders, especially preachers and schoolteachers.[41] Preachers were particularly important contacts because the church was generally the center of social activity for rural black communities. Preachers, many of whom performed agricultural labor themselves, could influence a community's response to the Movable School because of their respected social position. Uncooperative ministers could sabotage a program if they believed it interfered with their own work. Campbell remembered one time when a preacher told his congregation that the Tuskegee farm wagon was outside but that they "can't afford to engage in worldly affairs while we are busy engaged in saving souls, and I advise you not to take up any time with the wagon." With the preacher's closing warning about "silver tongued speakers," most of the people passed by the school.[42]

Other preachers lent their support to the educational program and led people in prayer during Movable School sessions. The extension agents tried to begin each session with "verses of scripture." One preacher offered his endorsement of the work of the school when he led those present in a prayer. According to Campbell's account, written to convey a southern black dialect, the preacher said: "O Lord, have mercy on this Removable School, may it pumernate [permeate] dis whole lan an country."[43]

No doubt some people rejected the idea of spending their spare time performing manual labor; however, for many the desire for education was so strong that they were drawn to the extension service programs. Agents documented numerous expressions of interest in the educational work of the Movable School. In Campbell's 1915 report he stated that a man spoke up one day after a Movable School demonstration and declared: "I aint no speaker but I jes wan'a tell you how much I has been steamilated [stimulated], this has been my two days in school."[44] In 1922 when agents held a demonstration on a large plantation they discovered that instead of teaching only one community, they had been teaching tenant farmers who had come from two areas where the school had just been. Many of the people had traveled ten to fifteen miles by foot and mule to attend the extra classes. A few years later Movable School nurse Eunice Rivers reported that she had met people who had already attended the school's classes but were coming again because "they were very anxious to hear the same lectures they had heard before."[45] The desire for entertainment as well as education may have motivated their return.

The rural black poor approached the arrival of extension agents in their communities with cautious interest. On the one hand, they were genuinely interested in education and improving their lot. On the other hand, they had reasons to be suspicious of outsiders, even those from the famous Tuskegee Institute. Based on previous experiences with local government and its history of upholding white supremacy, they were reluctant to participate in programs for fear of being exploited. They were also distrustful of the state and its representatives, given their mistreatment at the hands of landlords, courts, railroads, and law enforcement agents.[46]

Tenant farmers, and perhaps even the few black landowners, were wary of participating in programs that seemed to offer something for nothing, even when promoted by other black people. Campbell reported that some people doubted the truthfulness of agents' claims that the program was free, having been swindled too often by traveling salesmen.[47] Rural people were wary of outside interference, including that from government-sanctioned programs. "They would rather drink the worst kind of water than report to the state," observed home demonstration agent Laura Daly.[48] Once when Campbell was in Wilcox County talking to people to drum up support for a Movable School session, he raised the subject of the boll weevil. According to Campbell, a man in the audience rose and announced:

> Fesser, we sho enjoyed yo talk, but we naturally don't believe dere is any sich thing as a boll wesell. We bleve de store keepers and de fertilize fokes done paid you all to come out here and tell us bout dese bugs so as to make us work harder and buy more stuff fum dem.[49]

The rural poor may have had limited "book learning" but experience taught them to be on the lookout for exploitation.

Extension agents discovered that some of the rural people feared that agents were spying on them for white landowners. Possibly the greatest concern of tenant farmers and sharecroppers was to avoid injustice at the hands of white landlords. Many white plantation owners continued to treat the black people who worked for them as their own private property. Peonage, which was pervasive throughout the southern cotton belt in the early twentieth century, meant that some black farmworkers lived in what can only be called involuntary servitude. Landlords created peonage by using indebtedness to forbid sharecroppers to leave plantations, and they enforced it with the threat and reality of violence.[50]

Some farmworkers insisted that they would sign no formal agreements that might lock them into an oppressive relationship. Campbell remembered that after he had finished speaking at one meeting, a man from the audience stated:

> We is mighty glad to hab Dr. Washington to send you out to help us, but we don't see how he kin afford to give us free seed to plant our fields and pay you to come out here and see us once a month; so we thanks you fur your talk, but we can't sign no contract.[51]

The rural black poor had a realistic understanding of their situation and were not about to compound it by incurring additional expenses or obligations.

Black extension agents were very aware that they faced polite suspicion, if not always direct opposition, from rural black people wary of special schemes that promised much but frequently disappointed. One southern agricultural and mechanical school president warned those interested in black uplift work that "the underprivileged group for whom the program is planned must believe in it. Their suspicions of being exploited must be early allayed."[52] Black professionals knew that to reach black tenant farmers as well as the few landowners, they had to earn their trust.

The Limitations of Black Extension Service Work

Unable to alter the economic system in which rural black people lived, black professionals provided educational programs that offered advice on how to cope with the oppressive nature of the southern agricultural system. Yet, for black people who did not own their land or house, some of the instructions provided by the Movable School agents were impractical.[53] For many tenant farmers, perhaps most, there seemed little reason to fix up their homes because they had to move every year. Contemporary black sociologist Charles Johnson argued that changing residence, often within the same county, was tenant families' "one outstanding means of asserting freedom." Furthermore, some tenants found that landlords increased the rent after the tenants improved their place.[54]

The reports submitted by black extension agents with the Movable School indicated that they were aware of the limitations of their work. Born into tenant farm families themselves, they were not surprised by the living conditions they encountered; they presented shocking details of rural poverty to government officials in order to garner support. Campbell acknowledged that there was no use in painting a rosy picture of southern living to the rural black Southerner "who is constantly in debt, hungry, sick and cold, and without civil protection."[55] In 1922 George F. King observed that black reformers had to keep in mind the actual conditions of the people they wanted to assist:

> Many of the dilapidated shanties in which the Negroes live on plantations haven't windows . . . a mere space cut or made in the side of the house with shutters. . . . It is rather humorous to ask these poor people to sleep with their windows up without helping them to first make it possible to screen these openings. . . . We talk to the fellow out in the country who is up against conditions hard to describe at times about dieting or food values. Mighty good things to talk about, but thousands of these fellows are working under a system which keeps them from even raising a few collards — their gardens and pantries are the store of the owner of the plantation.[56]

It was difficult for black extension agents to alter systemic poverty through educational programs.

Furthermore, rural African Americans encountered alternative strategies for black advancement, including Marcus Garvey and the Universal Negro Improvement Association (UNIA), an international organization with millions of members in the early 1920s. This social movement, labeled a back-to-Africa movement, sought racial advancement through black separatism and an emphasis on black pride. Membership dues provided sickness and death benefits, and women created the Black Cross Nurses, a female auxiliary of the UNIA.[57] Often thought of as a northern, urban mass movement, the UNIA reached deep into the rural South.

Some white Southerners and government agricultural leaders feared that the black agricultural labor force would be attracted to the Garvey movement and leave the South for Africa. In 1923 the U.S. Department of Agriculture learned from a black extension agent's report that four farmers' clubs in his county in Alabama had folded and that

> this movement brought a great setback to these communities, as many of the farmers did nothing but walk around and talk about going to Africa and made no effort to progress as farmers. Not one of these farmers ever left, but they lost the year talking about it.[58]

For some African Americans the UNIA offered more attractive possibilities than the programs provided by extension service agents.

Black leaders, such as Campbell and Work, warned that poor health conditions, inadequate educational opportunities, and overall mistreatment were the primary causes of black migration and that until these improved, it would be difficult to slow the loss of black agricultural workers.[59] There was no mass exodus to Africa, but many black Southerners left the countryside.

Black extension agents had to negotiate a fine line between conforming to southern racial customs and advancing black rights. Despite his own belief that black people were entitled to programs, Campbell used white fear of black migration to argue for money to hire more black extension agents, suggesting that they were useful to stem black migration. In his public pronouncements, Campbell argued that black extension work benefited southern agriculture by making agricultural labor more profitable, productive, and pleasurable. He insisted that extension work improved race relations between black and white people "and above all, it is doing untold good towards gaining for the South an intelligent, peaceful and contented farm laborer."[60]

Even in statements that criticized poor living standards, black extension agents tried to illustrate the national significance of alleviating the distant poverty of the black sharecropper. For example, Campbell wrote that the shacks of rural black people "conveyed a generally bad impression of shiftlessness and backwardness." Yet he urged white America to take note of the living conditions of the black rural poor because "the squalor, filth, disease and dilapidation of their surroundings reflect not only upon them, but upon the whole South; and this condition constitutes not only a Negro problem, nor a Southern problem, but a national one."[61]

In 1921 the Extension Service of the U.S. Department of Agriculture made a film entitled *Helping Negroes to Become Better Farmers and Homemakers* to encourage rural African Americans to stay on the farm. Campbell, the Movable School, and Tuskegee Institute all appeared in this thirty-minute silent film made by the federal government in Macon County. The film told a fictional story of Rube and Hannah Collins, black tenant farmers who learned that they could prosper in the South with the help of the Extension Service. When Rube detected a boll weevil in the cotton, he properly notified his landlord, who called in the white extension agent to get rid of it. The film also depicted the arrival of the Movable School and people arriving from miles around to attend sessions, including one by a home demonstration agent who taught Hannah the proper way to set a table and one from a public health nurse on home nursing.

Black agents showed this government film regularly at sessions of the Movable School around the state. An agent used a film projector in the Movable School truck and directed it at a sheet pinned up on a cabin's outside wall. The rural people apparently enjoyed watching the film for the novelty of it and because they recognized Campbell and Tuskegee Institute.[62]

This film encapsulates some of the constraints on black extension work, which could do little to alter the oppressive conditions under which black tenants lived, including a rigid racial hierarchy. The film concludes with a scene that was supposed to convey the image of "happy darkies," as black people ate watermelon, danced, and sang to the strains of "Swanee River" on the phonograph. Black extension agents knew this was a white fantasy, not black reality, yet they were forced to work within a system that insisted on these myths or they risked being fired.[63]

Ironically, there was a tension in the work of extension service agents between a desire to introduce rural African Americans to the benefits of modern living and the agents' knowledge that the kind of transformation they sought was unrealistic given the persistent poverty of black Southerners. Despite their understanding of the larger economic picture, black extension agents preached unrealistic messages that suggested that wanting a better life would make it so. Home demonstration agent Daly explained the goal:

> The demonstration agents try to inspire the rural people "to want," to want more convenient, livable homes, more beautiful surroundings, to want health, education and to want, to a more appreciable degree, to enjoy the civilization in which they live.[64]

Ironically, such messages of modernization and consumer culture were also assertions of black entitlement and may have inspired some rural African Americans to leave in search of a better life.

The Movable School and Health Promotion: The Public Health Nurse

Although extension agents, especially home demonstration agents, addressed health issues informally as part of their other duties, the addition of a public health nurse in 1920 marked the beginning of formal health work for the Movable School. Health concerns were integral to rural development work. Campbell hired Uva M. Hester, a Tuskegee graduate, to help members of the Movable School guard against disease, look after the health of the people who attended Movable School sessions, and inspect the sanitation of homes and farms. By 1923, after some lobbying, Tuskegee Institute began to receive $100 per month from the Alabama Department of Health to assist with the salary of a nurse for the Movable School. In the early 1920s federal matching grants from the Sheppard-Towner Act doubled the number of people who had access to nursing care in Alabama.[65]

Campbell recalled that he decided to hire a nurse because, as the school traveled from county to county, evidence mounted of pervasive ill-health among black people. Campbell wrote in his 1936 autobiography and history of the Movable School:

> The truth of the matter is, we seriously considered abandoning the practice of going into the homes because of the constant danger and exposure of our workers to diseases and unsanitary conditions which we found in these homes. Being, however, so thoroughly conversant with this standard of living and so recently emerged from a similar atmosphere, I felt confident that these people were susceptible to the practical teaching we were taking to them. Instead of quitting the homes and returning to the public meeting places to conduct the schools, I sought the appointment of a registered nurse as a member of the Movable School force.[66]

Thus nursing came to the traveling school as protection for the extension workers, with the added benefit that they could visit rural clients.

Not everyone supported the inclusion of a nurse in the Movable School. Campbell reported that some physicians and nurses initially objected to the idea of a nurse traveling with the school and "predicted many difficulties and dangers that failed to develop."[67] They may have been concerned about the responses of local, mostly white, physicians who would have resisted encroachment on their private practice. To address this issue, Campbell suggested that the Alabama Department of Health explain to physicians the nature of the nurse's work with the school. He argued that

> if this nurse goes out and begins to give advice and the local doctor finds out and does not understand what it's all about he's going to raise a complaint. But if the State Health Department understands and passes the word to county units that this nurse is working for the State everything works fine.[68]

Like most public health nurses, Hester did not provide medical treatment but rather focused on health education, along with advice and care for the sick. She worked primarily with midwives and mothers, those in charge of family health care. She was supposed to instruct women in how to care for their children and sick family members, teach midwives how to ensure safe deliveries, and discourage the practice of folk medicine, such as using herbs and roots to treat illnesses.[69] Hester also distributed state health department literature, gave talks to parents about the care of children, and lectured schoolteachers on how to handle playground accidents.

Hester found the health conditions of rural families simply unbearable because of the unsanitary state of many homes. In her reports she indicated how appalled she was by the flies, the dirt, and the small rooms in the cabins she visited.[70] Her first week's report chronicled the inadequate health services available in rural Alabama:

> Tuesday: I visited a young woman who had been bedridden with tuberculosis for more than a year. There are two openings on her chest and one in the side from which pus constantly streams. In addition, there is a bedsore on the lower part of the back as large as one's hand. There were no sheets on her bed. . . . The sores had only a patch of cloth plastered over them. No effort was made to protect the patient from the flies that swarmed around her.[71]

These same themes of unhealthy conditions and inadequate bedside care recur frequently in Hester's reports from her travels throughout the county.

As a public health nurse, Hester was in an excellent position to assess the health needs of rural African Americans, but she could do little to provide medical treatment. Instead, she provided health education and comfort where she could. While traveling in Pickett Springs, for example, Hester saw a young girl with intestinal hemorrhages who needed medical attention. The house was dirty and there were no screens on the windows to stop the flies from coming in from the cow pen in the backyard. Hester reported:

> With my limited time there was little I could do to make her comfortable, however, I made a few suggestions as to diet, made her bed and tried to impress the importance of keeping out flies.[72]

In Capitol Heights, Hester discovered a seventeen-year-old girl who had undergone an operation in a hospital for abscesses on the chest and side. Hester explained:

> I found her lying in a bed of wheat straw, too filthy for description, with a profuse discharge of pus from these undressed wounds. The flies were over her in such numbers that I could hardly see her face, and she with a branch from a tree was making a feeble attempt to keep them off. There was an old cot on the little porch, so I suggested that we make it as comfortable as possible and put her on it. We did. I gave her a bath and while doing so I found she had a pressure sore on the sacral region of her back, the size of my hand, with backbone protruding. I dressed the wound with material from my first aid bag.[73]

The girl thanked Hester with tears in her eyes and told the nurse that, if she could, she would ask her grandmother to give Hester a pig for all her help.

Mary E. Williams from Virginia served as the next Movable School Nurse in early 1922 until she became head of the new Tuskegee Institute Health Center that September.[74] Williams inspected the sanitation of churches and schools and gave health lectures to children, including toothbrushing drills. She taught women home nursing techniques, including how to prevent bed sores, provide bed baths, make mustard plasters and poultices, provide proper ventilation, and eliminate the dangers of flies and mosquitoes. In April 1922 Williams reported that "most of the homes visited are very humble and the people very appreciative."[75]

Then in January 1923, Campbell hired nurse Eunice Rivers to work with the Movable School. Rivers (1899–1986), like most who worked with the school, had attended Tuskegee Institute and graduated from the nursing school in 1922. Born in rural Georgia, she was the oldest of three daughters of a farming family. Rivers became a nurse because of parental encouragement. She remembered that, before her mother died when Rivers was only fifteen, her mother had told her to "get a good education, so that I wouldn't have to work in the fields so hard." Her father also promoted education for his daughters, working long hours in a sawmill to help finance it. Rivers eventually followed her father's advice to study nursing despite protesting, "but Papa, I don't want to be no nurse, I don't want folks dying on me."[76] Rivers secured the position with the Movable School after caring for Monroe Work's sick wife Florence.[77] Like Hester and Williams before her, Eunice Rivers traveled in the Movable School truck with the home demonstration agent and the farm agent.

Gender prescriptions influenced the shape of Rivers's public health work as she traveled from county to county. She directed most of her health education messages, including discussion of sanitation, ventilation, and cleanliness, to rural women. Rivers informed women about specific diseases, such as malaria and typhoid fever, and taught them how to make bandages from old clothes, care for bedridden patients, and take a temperature. Women often asked questions at these health meetings and seemed eager for information. In addition, Rivers gave dental hygiene lectures to children on how to brush their teeth, and she handed out tubes of Colgate toothpaste donated by the company. Her public health work with men focused on "social hygiene," which usually meant information about the dangers of venereal disease.[78]

Rural women incorporated the free services of the public health nurse into their existing informal health care system of midwives and home remedies. They increasingly turned to nurses for advice, even as nurses tried to convince people to use physicians more often. Black people were hesitant to call on rural doctors, most of whom were white, because the doctors often did not treat them with respect and because many required payment in cash.

Even when African-American health institutions and workers were available, at least some rural people were hesitant to use them. Home demonstration agent Laura Daly detected a fear of doctors and hospitals among rural women attending the 1930 commencement exercises at Tuskegee Institute. When asked to leave their babies with nurses in the hospital, "some expressed fear less the doctors use their babies for experiments or something like that, [while] others were made afraid by the idea of a hospital."[79]

In 1926 Rivers redirected some of the focus of her public health work toward reproductive health. The state transferred her from the Alabama Bureau of Child Welfare, in which she performed her Movable School work, to the Bureau of Vital Statistics. Her new mandate was to assist the state in creating a system of registration for births and deaths, as well as aid efforts to regulate lay midwifery and lower infant mortality rates. She continued to travel throughout Alabama with the Movable School, but she focused her attention on pregnant women and midwives.[80]

Rivers was well-liked, and the people apparently appreciated her visits. She reached many people through her Movable School position and worked in over twenty counties in her first year alone. She visited hundreds of people every month; during one particularly busy month she tended to 1,100 people. J. D. Barnes, a white extension agent in Greene County, reported to Tuskegee Institute in 1928 that rural women remembered Rivers's visits and the way she made people feel good in her company. He wrote, "one woman asked me when I was going to have that sweet little woman come back to the county again."[81] Despite contracting malaria one month while on her rounds, she maintained a steady pace of presenting public health programs and attending national conferences of public health nurses, extension service agents, and teachers.[82]

Rivers, who grew up with a class background similar to that of the people she treated, attributed her successful relationships with rural people to her attitude toward them. "As far as I was concerned," she explained, "every individual was an individual of his own. He didn't come in a lump sum." She remembered that sometimes people would ask her how she ever received entry into certain homes where visitors were not welcomed. Rivers would reply:

> Well, darling, I don't know. I was brought in there. They're people as far as I'm concerned. I don't go there dogging them about keeping the house clean. I go there and visit a while until I know when to make some suggestions. When I go to the house I accept the house as I find it. I bide my time.[83]

Her approach, she concluded, was nothing more than mutual respect between herself and those she assisted. The degree of trust and the close relationships that she developed with rural African Americans through her work with the Movable School proved to be a tremendous asset in her work for the USPHS.

Bad Blood in Alabama: The Tuskegee Syphilis Experiment

In 1932 Rivers, along with leaders of Tuskegee Institute, became involved with a study by the USPHS that appears to contradict her efforts to improve black health through the Tuskegee Movable School. Rivers's need for employment, as well as her interest in black health conditions, influenced her decision to accept employment with the USPHS. During the early 1930s, financial cutbacks caused by the onset of the Depression ended her job with the Movable School. Facing unemployment, she accepted a job as night supervisor at the John A. Andrew Memorial Hospital at Tuskegee Institute and worked there eight months until she learned of the position with the federal government. Campbell and Dr. Eugene Dibble recommended her for the job. When asked in later years why she went to work with the Syphilis Study she replied: "I was just interested. I mean I wanted to get into everything that I possibly could."[84] An equally compelling reason, no doubt, was her statement: "I was so glad to go off night duty that I would have done anything."[85] Thereafter, Rivers worked part-time for the USPHS and part-time in maternal and child health for Tuskegee's hospital and then later for the county health department.

Although historians have noted the key role that Rivers played in the experiment, they have presented her as a victim by virtue of her status as a woman, an African American, and a nurse. Groundbreaking work by James Jones, for example, interpreted much of Rivers's participation as driven by obedience to higher authority. A more satisfactory consideration of her role as an historical subject is in order; yet, examination of Rivers's role does not necessarily lead to an interpretation of her as an evil nurse. What does it mean, then, to talk about the historical agency of black women within racist and sexist social structures? Indeed, Rivers was neither a victim nor a villain but a complex figure who can only be understood within her historical context. She acted in ways she determined to be in her best interests and in the interests of promoting black health. Consistent with the responses of at least some black health professionals and educators at the time, Rivers did not question the experiment because she did not find it objectionable.

VENEREAL DISEASE CONTROL AND BLACK COMMUNITIES

In the early twentieth century, private foundations and the federal government focused attention on controlling venereal disease. The USPHS first addressed the topic of venereal disease during World War I when the government became concerned about the results of tests of military recruits that showed that many men, black and white, were infected with syphilis. The USPHS formed the Division of Venereal Disease to promote health education in black and white communities.[86] In the late 1920s the Julius Rosenwald Fund, with its strong interest in health care for African Americans,

assisted the USPHS in venereal disease control work. The foundation provided financial support to develop a demonstration control program for
African Americans in the South. This project to detect and treat syphilis
began in 1928 in Bolivar County, Mississippi, among thousands of black
tenant farmers and sharecroppers, and it appeared to show that nearly 20
percent of the men and women had syphilis. The Rosenwald Fund next expanded the program from Mississippi to counties in other southern states,
including Macon County in Alabama.[87] In 1932, when the Depression led
the Rosenwald Fund to discontinue its financial support, leaders of the
USPHS launched the Tuskegee Syphilis Study in Alabama. Initially, the
study was to continue for about six to twelve months.

White assumptions about the health and sexuality of African Americans influenced the way medical authorities interpreted statistical data on
venereal disease. Some black leaders criticized the high syphilitic rate always
cited for African Americans as well as the expectation that syphilis was
endemic to black populations because of sexual promiscuity. For example,
Dr. Louis T. Wright, a leader of the National Association for the Advancement of Colored People (NAACP), wrote that even if there were high rates
"this is not due to lack of morals, but more directly to lack of money, since
with adequate funds these diseases can be controlled easily."[88]

Confident that racial differences affected health and disease, white physicians of the USPHS expected the Tuskegee study to provide a useful racial
comparison to an Oslo study that traced untreated syphilis in Norway.
However, the Oslo study was a *retrospective* study examining previous case
records of white people whose syphilis went untreated, unlike the Tuskegee
study, which was designed to deliberately withhold available treatment
from black people. Dr. Raymond Vonderlehr, an official at the USPHS,
even proposed that they expand their investigation, suggesting that "similar
studies of untreated syphilis in other racial groups might also be arranged."
He proposed that they conduct a study of Native Americans with untreated
syphilis.[89]

BLACK PROFESSIONALS STRIKE A BARGAIN
Black leaders at Tuskegee Institute endorsed the government study, to the
relief of the federal officials, in the belief that it would help the school in
its work for African Americans. The government doctors selected Macon
County because they had identified it as having the highest rate of syphilis
of all the Rosenwald study groups, with a rate of about 35 percent, and because they rightly concluded that Tuskegee Institute could provide valuable

assistance. Dibble, the medical director of Tuskegee's hospital, supported the experiment on the grounds that it might demonstrate that costly treatment was unnecessary for people who had latent or third-stage syphilis, echoing the justifications provided by the USPHS. More importantly, Dibble urged Moton to support the study because Tuskegee Institute "would get credit for this piece of research work," and the study would "add greatly to the educational advantages offered our interns and nurses as well as the added standing it will give the hospital." Moton agreed to allow the school's employees to examine the men in the study at Tuskegee's Andrew Hospital. Apparently, he believed that federal attention to the poor health conditions in the county would help the school get more funding for programs.[90]

Like the advantages of government aid to the Movable School, black educators and doctors at Tuskegee envisioned future financial benefits from cooperating with the federal government in the study. Such a belief grew out of Tuskegee's long history of lobbying the federal government for funding and assistance. Since the days of Booker T. Washington, black leaders at Tuskegee had witnessed evidence of at least limited government cooperation. For example, Washington and, later, Moton garnered government support for the Movable School and the National Negro Health Movement and succeeded in getting a black veterans' hospital located at Tuskegee, despite the absence of a black medical school.[91]

The experiment, officially known as "the Tuskegee Study of Untreated Syphilis in the Negro Male," was not a government secret, kept hidden from health professionals. It lasted for forty years and was publicized widely in the black and white medical community without evoking any protest. In the mid-1930s Dr. Roscoe C. Brown, as head of the Office of Negro Health Work at the USPHS, convinced the National Medical Association (NMA) to display an exhibit on the study provided by the government. Brown argued that it "would be an excellent opportunity for the use of this timely exhibit on one of our major health problems."[92] Members of the black medical establishment knew the subjects of the experiment were poor black men, but they did not see this as problematic. Not until 1973, after a journalist broke the story to the general public, did the black medical establishment denounce the study as morally, ethically, and scientifically unjustified. By then, a civil rights movement and a popular health movement critical of medicine resulted in an atmosphere of changed consciousness about rights and responsibilities.[93]

Why did black professionals, including Rivers, not challenge the study? Dr. Paul B. Cornely of Howard University, a black public health leader since the 1930s, remembered with regret that he knew about the experiment from the beginning. He understood the nature of the study and had followed it all along, never questioning it. He explained in retrospect: "I was there and I didn't say a word. I saw it as an academician. It shows you how we looked at human beings, especially blacks who were expendable." Cornely taught about the study in his classes at Howard University Medical School, a black college in Washington, D.C., yet no student ever raised a challenge to what he now sees as its racist premise. Cornely asked himself why he did not see the full ramifications of the project. "I have guilt feelings about it, as I view it now," he explained, "because I considered myself to be an activist. I used to get hot and bothered about injustice and inequity, yet here right under my nose something is happening and I'm blind."[94]

No doubt a number of factors contributed to the response of black professionals, including class consciousness and professional status within black America, and racial subordination in relation to white America. Historian Tom W. Shick argued that the black medical profession did not challenge the experiment because "black physicians were clearly subordinates, never co-equals, within the medical profession." Furthermore, he believed that the process of professionalization in medicine led them to defend the status quo. James Jones stated that class consciousness permitted black professionals to deny the racism of the experiment.[95]

Although subordinate status no doubt constrained the response of black professionals, they did not protest the syphilis study because they did not view it as unjust. Indeed, black educators and health professionals supported the study because they saw it directing federal attention toward black health problems—a primary goal of the black public health movement. As far as they were concerned, this was a study that focused the objective gaze of science on the health conditions of African Americans. It was one more way to increase the visibility of black needs to the federal government. Rivers shared the viewpoint of black health professionals and assisted with the experiment in the belief that the study was itself a sign of government interest in black health problems.

BLACK TENANT FARMERS IN SEARCH OF HEALTH CARE

Why, despite a history of well-founded suspicion of government, did black tenant farmers take part in the government study? The answer lies in the impact of the work performed in Macon County by Tuskegee Institute, the Movable School, and Rivers. The experiment began in October 1932 as Rivers assisted the USPHS in recruiting and testing rural black people in the county for syphilis so physicians could identify candidates for the study. Rivers was familiar with this work because she had assisted with the earlier syphilis treatment project sponsored by the Rosenwald Fund. Most likely her presence contributed to local interest in the clinics; Rivers and the government physicians were overwhelmed by the number of people who showed up at the sites to have their blood tested and receive treatments.[96] One man was even unhappy about his diagnosis: "They said my blood was good. You don't get no treatment if your blood is good, but sometimes I wish it was bad 'cause they gives away a salve up there and I wanted some of it so bad."[97]

Equal numbers of women and men appeared at the clinic sites, which proved to be a problem because the government doctors had decided to study only men. Dr. Joseph Earle Moore of Johns Hopkins University School of Medicine suggested the study focus on men because, he argued, women's symptoms of syphilis at the early stage were usually mild, and it was more difficult for physicians to examine internal organs.[98] Yet, as much as the doctors and Rivers tried to test only men, women showed up at the clinics too. Attempts to segregate the men led to new problems. According to Dr. Vonderlehr, "In trying to get a larger number of men in the primary surveys during December we were accused in one community of examining prospective recruits for the Army."[99] Rivers reported that some of the women, especially the wives of the men selected for the study, were mad that they were not included because "they were sick too." Some even told her, "Nurse Rivers, you just partial to the men."[100]

Jones cited Charles Johnson's 1934 investigation of African Americans in Macon County as evidence that poor African Americans participated in the study because of their tradition of dependence and obedience to authority.[101] Yet, Jones's own work suggests that poor African Americans in fact questioned authority, including that of white physicians. For example, Jones described one man who criticized the way a government doctor drew blood samples and recounted how "he lay our arm down like he guttin' a hog." The man reported: "I told him he hurt me. . . . He told me 'I'm the doctor.' I told him all right but this my arm."[102] Rivers remembered that sometimes the young white doctors would behave rudely toward the men and the men would ask her to intervene. A man told her once: "Mrs. Rivers, go in there and tell that white man to stop talking to us like that." So she went in and said: "Now, we don't talk to our patients like this. . . . They're human. You don't talk to them like that." The doctor even apologized.[103]

Rural African Americans cooperated not out of deference to white doctors but because they wanted medical attention and treatment for their ailments, and they had come to trust Rivers as someone who helped them. Even though the government doctors in the study changed over the years, Rivers provided the continuity. Without her assistance it is doubtful that the experiment would have been able to continue for so long with such cooperation from the subjects of the experiment. In addition, participating in the study gave these tenant farmers increased status as they gained an official association with both the prestigious Tuskegee Institute and the federal government, relationships typically unavailable to men of their class.

The men stayed with the study for forty years because they believed they received something worthwhile. Rivers found that the men who joined the study "had all kinds of complaints" about what ailed them, and they continued with the study in order to get free treatments. However, the men joined under false pretenses because the health workers never informed the men that they had syphilis or that they would not receive treatment. Instead, the men were told they would be treated for "bad blood," a vague term that referred to a range of ailments, including general malaise. The men were not told that they could spread the disease to their sexual partners or that they were part of an experiment predicated on nontreatment of syphilis until death. What the USPHS provided was annual physical examinations, aspirin, free hot meals on the day the government physicians visited, and financial support for burial expenses. In a rural community where there was almost no formal health care available, and if poor black people could locate it they could not afford it, these limited benefits were desirable and convinced the men to continue in the study.[104]

NURSE EUNICE RIVERS AND GOVERNMENT PUBLIC HEALTH WORK

As for Eunice Rivers, what motivated her to work for the experiment for so many years? Historians have argued that Rivers participated because (1) she could not have understood the full ramifications of the study, and (2) as a black female nurse she was in no position to challenge the authority of white male physicians.[105] Evidence suggests, however, that Rivers had sufficient knowledge of the study to know that the men were systematically denied treatment. In fact, Rivers was one of the authors, listed first, of a follow-up paper about the study published in 1953 in *Public Health Reports*. Rivers had published on public health work before, in a 1926 report on her work with the Movable School in *Public Health Nurse*.[106]

However, even if Rivers herself did not write the report, which read like a tribute to her role in the study, her actions made clear that she was

well aware of the terms of the experiment. After all, she was one of the
people who helped to implement the policy, designed by the leaders of the
USPHS, to prohibit the subjects of the study from receiving treatments for
syphilis from anyone else. This meant denying the treatment available during the 1930s and the penicillin available after World War II. At the same
time that Rivers assisted with the treatment of syphilis in other public
health programs, she helped carry out the experiment's plan to bar the men
in the government study from treatment.[107]

Finally, based upon how Rivers operated as a nurse, suggestions that
she merely deferred to authority are not convincing. She no doubt knew
how to tailor her comments and behavior to a given situation to preserve
her position and dignity. However, despite the racial, gender, and medical
hierarchies under which she operated, she saw herself as an advocate for her
patients and acted accordingly. She did not hesitate to intervene on their
behalf, even consulting one doctor when she questioned the procedures of
another.

If ignorance and deference do not explain her behavior, what does?
Her need for employment and the prestige of working for the federal government certainly contributed to her participation. She was proud of her
work, and the federal government honored her for assistance in the experiment. For example, in 1958 she received an award from the Department of
Health, Education and Welfare "for an outstanding contribution to health,
through her participation in the long-term study of venereal disease control
in Macon County, Alabama."[108]

Most importantly, Rivers considered her participation in the study
merely a continuation of her previous public health work. Public health
work was gendered to the extent that women, especially in their capacity as
nurses, implemented health policy and had the most contact with people in
the community. In Rivers's case, since the early 1920s her job had been to
provide health education directly to people in the communities surrounding Tuskegee. Her duty as a nurse was to care for her clients, and she did. In
her work with the experiment, she developed close relationships with the
men. One of the government physicians even told her that she was too
sympathetic with the men. As Rivers explained: "I was concerned about the
patients 'cause I had to live here after he was gone." Indeed, she knew each
man individually and, after he died, she attended the funeral service with
the man's family. "I was expected to be there," she recalled, "they were part
of my family."[109] In nominating Rivers for an award in 1972, Thelma P.
Walker revealed that Rivers "has been my inspiration for entering public
health. She made her own work so attractive because of her enthusiasm. . . .

She inspired such confidence in her patients and they all seem so endeared to her." Walker discovered "how deeply loved she was by the men in her follow-up program. They felt that there just was no one like Mrs. Rivers."[110]

When the press exposed the study in 1972, it was confusing and heart-breaking for Rivers to hear the criticism after having received so much praise. Rivers responded by defending her actions. "A lot of things that have been written have been unfair," she insisted. "A lot of things."

First, Rivers argued that the effects of the experiment were benign. In her mind it was important that the study did not include people who had early syphilis because those with latent syphilis were potentially less infectious and would be less likely to transmit it to their sexual partners. As she explained, "syphilis had done its damage with most of the people."[111] Yet, as historian Allan Brandt noted, "every major textbook of syphilis at the time of the Tuskegee Study's inception strongly advocated treating syphilis even in its latent stages."[112]

Second, Rivers accounted for her participation by stating that the study had scientific merit. Even as she admitted, "I got with this syphilitic program that was sort of a hoodwink thing, I suppose," she offered justification. With great exaggeration, she depicted Macon County as "overrun with syphilis and gonorrhea. In fact, the rate of syphilis in the Negro was very, very high, something like eighty percent or something like this."[113] She recalled that the government doctors planned to compare the results of the study with one in Norway on white people and that "the doctors themselves have said that the study has proven that syphilis did not affect the Negro as it did the white man."[114]

Finally, based on the available health care resources, Rivers believed that the benefits of the study to the men outweighed the risks. Rivers knew the men received no treatment for syphilis, but she explained:

> Honestly, those people got all kinds of examinations and medical care that they never would have gotten. I've taken them over to the hospital and they'd have a GI series on them, the heart, the lung, just everything. It was just impossible for just an ordinary person to get that kind of examination.[115]

She continually asserted that the men received good medical care despite the fact that the men received mostly diagnostic, not curative, services. Yet she maintained

> they'd get all kinds of extra things, cardiograms and . . . some of the things that I had never heard of. This is the thing that really hurt me about the unfair publicity. Those people had been given better care than some of us who could afford it.[116]

What bothered Rivers was not the plight of the men in the study but that of the women and men who came to her begging to be included, even leading her occasionally to sneak in some additional men. As for the men in the experiment, Rivers concluded that they received more, not less, than those around them: "They didn't get treatment for syphilis, but they got so much else."[117]

Conclusion

Racism, extreme poverty, and health care deprivation in rural Alabama, where so little medical attention could mean so much, contributed to a situation in which white doctors from the federal government could carry out such an experiment on African Americans with the assistance of black professionals. Rivers as well as health workers and educators from Tuskegee Institute, Howard University, and the NMA never challenged the study because they believed that it was an acceptable way to gather knowledge. It seems that Rivers and other black professionals shared the dominant vision of scientific research and medical practice and did not consider issues of informed consent. Perhaps professionalization and class consciousness blinded them to the high price paid by the poor, rural black men in the study.[118]

Furthermore, the gendered nature of public health work meant that the nurse, invariably a woman, was at the center of public provisions, both the good and the bad. Thus, the role of Eunice Rivers in the experiment has drawn particular attention. After public censure forced the halt of the experiment, Rivers declared her innocence in the face of criticism, not on the grounds that she was a victim who was uniformed about the true nature of the experiment but rather because she insisted that she had acted on her convictions. She emphasized:

> I don't have any regrets. You can't regret doing what you did when you knew you were doing right. I know from my personal feelings how I felt. I feel I did good in working with the people. I know I didn't mislead anyone.[119]

Rivers remained convinced that she had acted in the best interests of poor black people.

As the actions of Eunice Rivers show most starkly, the constraints on black health reform led black professionals to strike a risky bargain with the federal government in an attempt to advance black rights. Government involvement generally proved to be advantageous to black middle-class professionals, but not always to the poor. Class status affected the price paid by African Americans when the government proved to be an untrustworthy ally. In the Tuskegee Movable School, where Tuskegee Institute ran the program despite a degree of federal funding, the benefits outweighed the costs to the poor. However, in the Tuskegee Syphilis Study where the USPHS controlled the agenda, there were deadly consequences for the poor.

5. The Public Health Work of Poor Rural Women

Black Midwives in Mississippi

In contrast to the tragedy of the Tuskegee Syphilis Study, the history of midwifery indicates some of the ways that government intervention was reshaped by the black rural poor to the benefit of black community health. Black lay midwives used the opportunity provided by government regulation to become important health workers well beyond their midwifery practice. Midwives, who were often sharecroppers themselves, provided health services to poor rural women and children and health education to the entire community. They helped public health nurses promote clinics, immunization programs, and prenatal and postnatal medical examinations. The success of official state and county health projects for African Americans depended to a large degree on the public health work of black laywomen. Indeed, from 1920 to 1950 African-American midwives helped to implement the modern public health care system in Mississippi and other southern states.

Ironically, state intervention in the previously unregulated practice of midwifery led to the creation of an unexpected cadre of black public health workers. Midwives were unique among health workers in that they were simultaneously the targets and the purveyors of health reform. By 1920 government concern over high infant and maternal mortality rates led officials to identify midwives as a public health problem. Public health nurses and doctors claimed that midwives did not maintain clean environments and that they used unscientific, and therefore unsafe, folk medicine. In response, southern states such as Mississippi enacted restrictions on midwifery practice through midwife training programs and registration requirements. Records of the Mississippi State Board of Health, including public health nurses' reports and correspondence from midwives, depict an ambiguous relationship between the state and poor black women. Although public health officials continued to define midwives as at best a "necessary evil," midwives proved to be a vital link between poor African Americans and health departments.

The Midwives of Mississippi

Across the nation, lay midwives delivered half of all babies as late as 1910. Much of the practice was among European immigrant women and southern black women. By 1930, with immigration restrictions and the preference of urban women for childbirth attendance by physicians, midwives delivered only 15 percent of all births.[1] At that time, 80 percent of all remaining midwives practiced in the South, where most were African Americans. Even as midwifery declined in significance in northeastern and midwestern urban areas, the number of practicing midwives did not drop significantly in the South until after 1950.[2]

In Mississippi, where half the population was black, the vast majority of midwives were black women. During the 1920s and 1930s Mississippi officials registered about 4,000 black midwives and only a few hundred white.[3] Other southern states detected equal or greater numbers of practicing midwives, most of whom were black, including 3,000 in Alabama, 5,000 to 6,000 in Georgia, 4,000 to 9,000 in North Carolina, and perhaps as many as 10,000 in Florida. These figures are rough estimates because health officials had no definite idea of the number of unregistered midwives who delivered babies.[4]

Black midwives, often called "granny" midwives by white health officials and occasionally by themselves, delivered over 25 percent of all babies and over 50 percent of black babies throughout the South. In Mississippi they delivered 80 percent of black babies until well into the 1940s, although the percentage of white babies they delivered dropped from 8 percent in the 1920s to 5 percent in the 1940s. Midwives tended most of the black women and a few white women, while doctors cared for most of the white women and only rarely black women. In her own practice, Mississippi midwife Della Falkner recorded the delivery of 120 black and 13 white babies from 1926 to 1936.[5]

Although black midwives were part of the rural poor, they were highly prestigious members of the communities they served. They were respected health care experts and played an important role in cultural transmission and community leadership. Midwives, along with teachers, were the female counterparts to preachers as the most influential people in rural areas. They were at the center of traditional healing networks in black communities of the South and served as advisers and spiritual leaders.[6]

Southern black women, and some white ones, preferred midwife over physician deliveries for economic and cultural reasons. In general, midwives were cheaper than doctors and would more readily travel to remote places over rough roads. They provided comfort and support to pregnant women before, during, and after delivery. They even looked after the cooking and cleaning, in addition to caring for the mother and newborn, gendered tasks that male doctors were reluctant to perform. Even when a doctor was available, women may have preferred delivery by another woman because of sexual propriety or because they considered birth a natural process, not a medical event. Furthermore, unlike at least some white doctors, midwives generally treated black birthing women with dignity rather than disregard. Alabama midwife Onnie Lee Logan recalled that, too often, white doctors did not treat black people like human beings and that they had little interest in delivering black babies.[7]

Midwifery was only part of the work performed by black midwives. Most of them also cared for their own families, tended crops in the fields, and worked as domestic servants or even teachers. For example, in her autobiography Logan described her work as a domestic servant for white families.[8] Nurses noted that at certain times of the year they had difficulty maintaining attendance for midwife training sessions because the women were busy with agricultural labor. In 1923 nurse Agnes B. Belser related: "I have had but one midwife meeting as they begged off because of the cotton picking season."[9] Nurse Louise James mentioned that her "greatest trouble in having a full attendance was caused by this season being cane grinding season and most all old women are used to skim cane syrup. Very often I had to go to the mill to get my entire class."[10]

Although midwifery itself was an extension of women's domestic work, not all women became midwives.[11] Black midwives usually explained that they were called to their work by God or a female relative. Many women stated that God called them through a vision or dream. Others indicated that they followed their own mothers or grandmothers into midwifery. Many times a midwife's first delivery occurred when she had to attend to a woman in labor in the absence of her midwife mother or grandmother. For example, Mississippi midwife Mittie Patterson, who practiced midwifery for 45 years, made her first delivery because a woman went into labor when her midwife mother was ill. To a certain degree, midwives controlled the recruitment of new practitioners by encouraging particular women to join them.[12]

In terms of payment, midwives as well as rural doctors generally accepted whatever patients offered them. Many women did not insist on any remuneration because they believed they did God's work. However, most received a few dollars or payment in kind, such as food or livestock. One woman in Alabama gave her cow, a substantial sacrifice, to the midwife for her delivery because her husband could not pay the fee in cash.[13] Bessie Sutton, who delivered her first baby in 1922, received about $1.50 for her deliveries in the 1920s, and when she retired in 1962 the fee had increased to $20. Early in this century northern immigrant and southern black women commonly received from one to five dollars for a delivery. Sutton explained that she did not do the work for the money but because she loved people. She emphasized, "if I'd a stopped 'cause they didn't pay me, I'd a stopped a long time ago."[14]

At least one midwife who did expect payment after a delivery grew quite impatient when it was late and took action into her own hands. In 1939 Mamie Reed of Leflore County delivered a baby,

> collected part of her fee and waited for the rest. After several weeks of waiting she requested the rest of the fee, and when refused took the baby as collateral. But officers in the county did not agree that Mamie had a lien on the youngster she helped pilot into the world, and promptly put the mid-wife in jail at Greenwood charged with kidnapping.[15]

Midwives may have ministered to the needs of the sick and the poor, but they were not completely self-sacrificing.

Nurses, Midwives, and State Regulation

Beginning in the early 1920s, southern states hired public health nurses to regulate midwives by means of funding from the federal government through the Sheppard-Towner Act, a creation of women's national lobbying efforts.[16] The Mississippi State Board of Health used Sheppard-Towner funding to register midwives and provide training classes. This state activity brought midwives, most of whom were black, and public health nurses, most of whom were white, into close contact. Midwives and nurses developed a reciprocal relationship in which midwives aided the work of nurses, even as nurses provided them with training (see Figures 5 and 6).

Government interest in the "midwife problem" shifted to the rural South, where most black midwives lived, due to fewer practicing midwives in the urban North and Midwest and the post-World War I expansion of

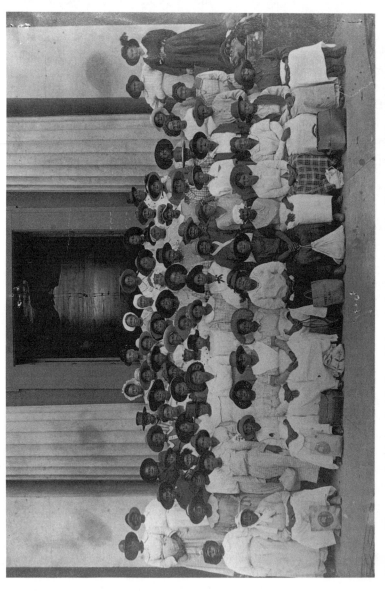

Figure 5. "A group of midwives in Madison County before any instruction." Courtesy of the Mississippi Department of Archives and History, Jackson, Mississippi.

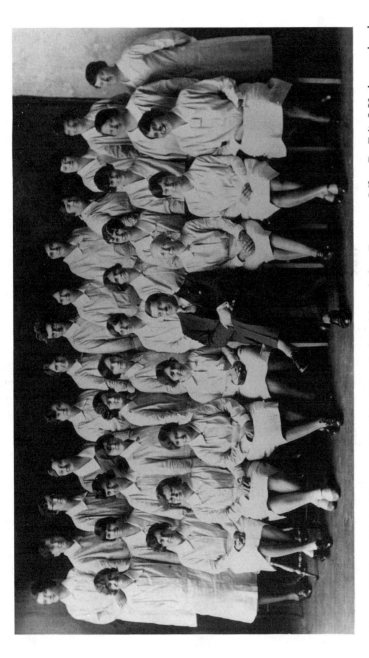

Figure 6. White public health nurses, Mississippi Board of Health, including Executive Officer Dr. Felix J. Underwood and Nursing Supervisor Mary D. Osborne (on his left), circa 1927. Courtesy of the Mississippi Department of Archives and History, Jackson, Mississippi.

public health nursing into rural areas.[17] In the search to improve the public's health, government officials and health professionals typically criticized the health provisions of midwives, a vulnerable population with little economic or political power, and rarely questioned the quality of care by physicians.

Targeting midwives was an easier solution for public health officials dealing with an impoverished rural population than challenging the medical establishment or altering the economic and living conditions that contributed to ill-health. In 1921 Laurie Jean Reid, a white nurse with the United States Public Health Service (USPHS), came to Mississippi to survey the midwives of the state. Reid traveled around the 82 counties of Mississippi, tracking down the names of midwives and registering the women county by county. In the process she identified over 4,000 midwives in Mississippi.[18] As she indicated to the white Mississippi State Medical Association, her purpose was to address the fact that the United States had higher infant and maternal mortality rates than many European countries. Reid declared that these rates were caused by poor health care for pregnant women from "careless physicians and by illiterate and ignorant midwives."[19] Sidestepping the issue of physician care, she proposed that the state eliminate those midwives who were too old to be educated, and register and train those who remained.

Health officials hoped to improve the safety of childbirth by limiting the practice of midwifery to normal deliveries only and making them more aseptic (free from infected matter). They perceived midwives as ignorant, unclean, and superstitious. They blamed midwives' unsanitary techniques and folk medicine for high infant and maternal mortality rates. By the late nineteenth century medical science came to understand that postpartum infections were caused by microorganisms entering the uterus, and therefore health officials felt it imperative to train midwives about the necessity for sterile conditions.[20]

Despite the fact that health officials blamed midwives for maternal and infant deaths, the midwife safety record was not any worse than that of physicians. Some contemporary studies even showed that maternal mortality rates were lowest where the percentage of midwife-attended births was highest.[21] In 1923 nurse supervisor Lois Trabert of Mississippi's Bureau of Child Welfare proclaimed: "I firmly believe that when we do get these midwives properly trained, in as far as that is possible, that they will do better and cleaner work than the average country doctor."[22]

The decision to regulate, and only occasionally to eliminate, midwives derived from the fact that southern rural areas had an inadequate number of practicing physicians to serve as the sole childbirth attendants. For poor rural women, midwives were available where physicians were not. Between 1920 and 1950 Mississippi had only 1,000 to 1,800 practicing physicians, less than 75 of whom were black, and well over twice that number of midwives. For rural African Americans, physician care was at best supplementary to that of midwives.[23]

From 1910 to 1930 health reformers and medical professionals engaged in a debate over the future of midwives. While many obstetricians argued for the immediate elimination of midwives, most public health officials argued that they were needed, even if only temporarily. Most public health doctors and nurses in Mississippi supported the gradual, not immediate, elimination of midwives because they believed that they were needed until there were enough hospitals and doctors to care for rural women.[24]

However, not all public health professionals in Mississippi supported state efforts to regulate midwives, and even supporters exhibited racial prejudice toward the women. Some private physicians and county health officers, doctors employed by the state board of health to oversee public health work in a given county, thought it was a waste of time. They did not think midwives could be educated in proper birthing techniques, and they did not want the state to sanction midwifery.[25] Furthermore, supporters of midwife training did not necessarily maintain a respectful opinion of midwives. For example, in 1925 Dr. Felix J. Underwood read a paper before the Southern Medical Association in which he described the black midwife as "filthy and ignorant and not far removed from the jungles of Africa, laden with its atmosphere of weird superstition and voodooism."[26]

Despite such sentiments, Underwood represented the more "progressive" of Mississippi's executive health officers, and he was active in state and national public health promotion for over three decades. The death of his mother in childbirth when he was ten motivated him to go into public health work. He earned his medical degree from the University of Tennessee in 1908 and then he returned to Mississippi, where he combined private practice with work as a county health officer. In 1921 Underwood went to work for the Mississippi State Board of Health at the Bureau of Child Hygiene and after a few years became the executive officer, serving from 1924 to 1958. During his career, Underwood was a health adviser to President Roosevelt's Committee on Economic Security, which produced the 1935 Social Security Act, and he served as president of the Mississippi

State Medical Association, the Southern Medical Association, and the American Public Health Association.[27]

MIDWIFE TRAINING PROGRAMS

Public health nurses were the government health professionals responsible for midwife training campaigns to "modernize" midwifery. By the mid-1930s the Mississippi State Board of Health employed 125 white and 6 black public health nurses.[28] Whether or not midwives abided by the new regulations, through nurses the state placed limitations on the health services midwives were entitled to perform during childbirth and in general.

The primary job of the public health nurse was education. As Edna Roberts, who served as state supervisor of nurses in Mississippi, explained: "We teach people. That's what the public health nurse has always done."[29] She remembered providing midwives with a type of women's health course, including information about sexual reproduction and female anatomy. Nurses often used visual aids, such as anatomical models and pictures, to convey the lessons to illiterate women. Since their primary purpose was positive instruction, nurses were not supposed to belittle harmless folk beliefs of midwives, such as putting a hatchet under the birthing bed to cut the pain. Instead, they were to pay attention to promoting an aseptic birthing room.[30]

From 1920 to 1950, public health nurses implemented southern health boards' educational programs using midwife manuals that carried virtually the same message for three decades.[31] Most southern states published midwife manuals. The lessons taught by the nurses emphasized limitations on midwives and the ultimate authority of doctors. Above all else, the two issues nurses focused on were the importance of cleanliness and calling on a physician when complications developed during a delivery.[32]

The emphasis on cleanliness extended to midwife clothing and equipment. Before state training began, midwives wore whatever they chose and carried the tools of their trade in an assortment of bags, such as flour sacks. Nurses permitted midwives to continue carrying midwife bags, but midwives had to upgrade them from flour sacks to black leather bags. Nurses instructed midwives to perform deliveries wearing a clean white dress, a white mask, and a white paper cap, which nurses taught them to make to keep their hair out of the way. The nurses also insisted that midwives keep their hands and nails clean.[33]

State boards of health in the North and South followed a similar pattern of midwife instruction.[34] Nurses forbade midwives to use any herbal remedies in their childbirth work. In order to prevent infections, nurses instructed midwives not to perform any digital examination of women during labor; only doctors were allowed to put their hands into the birth canal. If midwives followed this rule, they no doubt had difficulty identifying how far dilated a woman's cervix was and the progression of labor.

Public health officials, including those at the Mississippi State Board of Health, argued that training midwives did lower mortality rates. Underwood pointed to evidence of a decline in state maternal and infant mortality rates. Infant mortality rates (the number of deaths per 1,000 live births in the first year of life) dropped over the decades, from 68 in 1921 to 47 in 1942 for the state as a whole, and from 85 to 54 for black infants. A similar pattern held for maternal mortality rates, which dropped from 9 per 1,000 deliveries in 1921 to 4 in 1942, with black rates dropping from 12 in 1921 to 5 in 1942. Indeed, across the nation maternal mortality rates dropped by the 1940s and 1950s as better-trained doctors and midwives, improved prenatal care, and the availability of antibiotics improved women's chances of surviving childbirth.[35]

MIDWIFE CLUB MEETINGS

Beginning in the 1920s, Mississippi required midwives to have monthly club meetings at which they were to further their knowledge. Dressed in their white delivery outfits, the midwives were supposed to read from the state's midwife manual and discuss any delivery problems they encountered. Although public health nurses initially organized the local clubs, the midwives ran the meetings themselves. Each midwife club selected a leader or president and a secretary, and they were in charge of reporting the minutes of the meeting to the county public health nurse or, if there was none, to the state supervisor of midwives.[36]

The midwife leader had authority over the other members of the club. The leader was often one of the most literate women in the community. She helped others fill out birth certificates, ran inspection of the midwives' bags and fingernails, and handed out silver nitrate eyedrops to prevent blindness in newborns caused by passing through the birth canal of mothers with gonorrhea. The eyedrops, provided free by the state, proved to be a major incentive for midwives to attend club meetings. Midwives may have recognized the effectiveness of the drops or may have wanted them to differentiate themselves from midwives who were not registered with the state. According to health officials, the use of eyedrops dramatically decreased the number of cases of infection in the state from 346 in 1925 to 99 in 1933.[37]

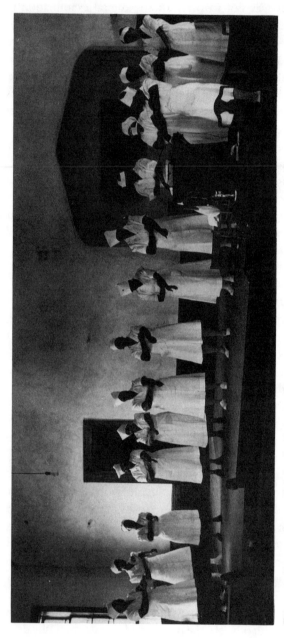

Figure 7. Forrest County Midwife Club demonstrating proper hygiene. Courtesy of the Mississippi Department of Archives and History, Jackson, Mississippi.

Midwife leaders ran the club meetings like a church service. Midwives usually held their meetings in churches, one of the few public buildings controlled by African Americans in rural communities. For example, the midwives of Hub, Mississippi met monthly at Sweet Valley Baptist Church.[38] At meetings, midwives had an opening prayer and song, read from the Bible and from "the Book" or midwife manual, and sang the midwife songs printed in the manual. Midwife songs included "Protect the Mother and Baby," sung to the tune of "Mary Had a Little Lamb," which had hand motions to go along with the lyrics describing the importance of clean clothes, clean hands, and clean midwives (see Figure 7).[39] In 1937 John Lomax, a native of Holmes County and curator of folk songs at the Library of Congress, recorded a dozen midwives singing such songs at the Mississippi State Board of Health.[40]

Even though midwives seemed to have enjoyed the opportunity to socialize with each other, share stories, and sing together, they could not always attend the monthly meetings. Attendance was down during times of heavy field labor and when weather made travel difficult, especially for women who had to walk several miles to the meetings. Despite the difficulty maintaining attendance, the number of midwife clubs increased over the years, growing from 290 clubs in the state in 1928 to 505 in 1942.[41]

MIDWIFE COMPLIANCE AND RESISTANCE TO STATE REGULATION

State regulation meant the creation of a division between state-sanctioned midwives and those midwives identified by the state as unfit to practice and therefore vulnerable to prosecution. Midwives both resisted and complied with various aspects of this state control. For example, the state enforced midwife registration through police power and the assistance of midwives themselves. In 1919 Ellen Woods Carter, a black nurse in lowcountry South Carolina, faced a group of midwives who refused to register, possibly because they had no interest or they feared state intrusion. They complied only after she "enlisted the services of the local registrar and the policeman to round up the group."[42] In other cases, registered midwives played a major role in the identification of unregistered midwives. In the 1920s the Mississippi State Board of Health located 1,000 unregistered midwives with the help of registered midwives. This assistance continued over the decades. For example, in 1939 a midwife club leader related to nurse Mary D. Osborne that Minerva P. of Jefferson County was practicing without a permit.[43]

Sometimes midwives used state regulation to gain advantages for themselves, such as setting standard fees. In 1944 a midwife club in Monroe County, under the leadership of midwives Sallie Mae Brock and Virginia Thompson, met at City Hall and voted to set a countywide fee for deliveries. They drew up resolutions that repeated state requirements and their decision to set a higher fee, stating the price was "to be fifteen dollars for the duration." They published their announcement in a local newspaper for a few weeks to inform all midwives in the county, concluding with the warning: "Now, if you feel you are unable to do this, just bring your permit to the City Hall and we will thank you."[44] Through this type of labor organizing, several midwives tried to get others to abide by the new fee or resign.

Midwives resisted state regulation when it conflicted with longstanding midwifery practices.[45] For example, nurses had difficultly convincing midwives to deliver women on the bed, not on the floor. Mothers and midwives particularly rejected this requirement because many women felt the urge to walk around during labor and found it more comfortable to deliver in a squatting position assisted by gravity instead of flat on their back in bed. Furthermore, some midwives preferred to keep the bed clean and have all the mess on the floor.[46] Alabama midwife Margaret Smith explained why she ignored the rule. As she pointed out, "when you in misery, if there is any way you can ease that misery, you gonna ease it."[47]

In order to ensure compliance with the rules, nurses occasionally supervised deliveries and inspected midwife bags. However, some midwives chose not to cooperate. Former county health officer Dr. W. E. Riecken, Jr., recalled that some midwives engaged in the practice of "a bag to show and a bag to go." Midwives used this strategy to circumvent the rules when they kept "a clean, properly organized bag for inspection and licensing and had another that was used for deliveries."[48] Nurse Elsie Davis mentioned in 1931 that some of the midwives with whom she worked refused to bring their bags for inspection, while others did not maintain their bags in sterile condition, offering the excuse that they just came off duty.[49] Nurses even inspected the homes of midwives to see that they understood the principles of cleanliness. Nurses Abbie G. Hall and Caroline Bourg of Sharkey-Issaquena counties reported: "We try to always keep in mind our midwives and never miss an opportunity to stop at their homes and inspect bags whenever we are in the neighborhood."[50]

Most midwives resented nurses' implications that they had not performed their work well before regulation by the state. They asserted that experience had already taught them the skills of midwifery. As midwife Otha Bell Jones of Itta Bena reported in 1938, she had learned how to be a midwife twenty-three years ago through apprenticing with midwife Nancy Wright, long before the existence of training programs. "And dear friends," she wrote the board of health, "I had nursed 36 womens before I got any permit and I has fill the sum of 15 books with 25 leaves each." Despite her long list of women she had delivered, she wrote: "[I] never lose a woman in childbirth since I have started out."[51] Midwife Onnie Lee Logan attended midwife training classes, but she emphasized that "two-thirds of what I know about deliverin, carin for mother and baby, what to expect, what was happenin and was goin on, I didn't get it from the class. God gave it to me. So many things I got from my own plain motherwit."[52] However, another midwife conceded that even though she had a great deal of knowledge, she could still learn more. "Each time I attend my monthly meeting I learn something new, and I am happy to admit that because so many won't."[53]

Midwives had a stake in convincing the state that they followed the regulations, even if in some aspects of their practice they did not. For example, in 1945 Mississippi midwife Georgette Smith contacted the state supervisor of midwives to let her know that she had married, changed her last name, and moved. Smith concluded her letter by stating: "Just want to Let you know Because i want to do rite and what the State say do."[54]

Midwives were cautious because the state threatened to revoke the permits of women who failed to follow the regulations. In 1923 Mississippi nurse Mae Reeves indicated that some nurses "found one midwife treating gynecological cases and children. We revoked her permit."[55] In 1924 a nurse in Washington County stated: "In follow up work for midwives found that one had delivered case without cap and gown, and had also made [digital] examination. Her permit was revoked for one month and at the end of that month she is not to take a case unless I can be with her at time of delivery."[56] Punishment for performing digital exams and failing to wear regulation uniforms could be swift. When one nurse revoked the permit of a midwife at a conference for the renewal of permits, the nurse realized that it "was so upsetting to the midwife that long wailing sobs penetrated the air. The sympathy of the other 75 midwives brought on more sobbing—needless to say I wondered just what I'd do to restore order and continue with the meeting."[57]

A midwife could also lose her permit if she performed abortions. Recent work by Leslie J. Reagan has demonstrated how the identification of midwives with abortion in Chicago in the early twentieth century paved the way for the regulation of immigrant midwives.[58] Although historians have discovered that some immigrant midwives met women's demands for abortions, there is almost no historical literature on black midwives and abortion. In 1950 Dr. James H. Ferguson of the Department of Obstetrics at Tulane University, New Orleans, suggested that "the less sophisticated rural midwife never acquired the reputation of abortionist as did her urban sister."[59] Debra Anne Susie, in her work on black midwives in Florida, has suggested that black midwives in the state did not perform abortions, or more accurately, the women she interviewed did not tell her that they ever performed abortions.[60] In Ruth C. Schaffer's study of black midwives in Texas, none of the women indicated that they performed abortions, even though 135 other interviewees stated that midwives did.[61]

Some black midwives did induce miscarriages; however, they may have been difficult for the state to detect. Midwife Logan indicated that although women asked her to do abortions, she never did them. Yet she remembered a midwife, her husband's grandmother, who performed abortions by inducing miscarriages. She remembered that the Alabama board of health suspected that some of the midwives deliberately caused miscarriages and revoked their permits.[62] The issue of abortion was strikingly absent in the board of health records in Mississippi. Retired nurse Edna Roberts believed that most midwives in the state did not perform abortions, but she indicated that if a nurse caught a midwife performing abortions the woman would lose her permit.[63]

Furthermore, midwives had their permits temporarily revoked if they tested positive for syphilis, the disease health officials were convinced was endemic to black America. In a parallel fashion, domestic servants were also required to be tested for syphilis. Nurses kept watch over midwives' health, fearful that midwives would spread diseases to birthing women and infants, much like health authorities feared disease transmission from domestics. The nurse required the midwife to have a Wassermann test for syphilis and vaccine against typhoid fever and smallpox.[64] Nurses administered Wassermann tests before they renewed permits each year, and nurses forbade midwives who had syphilis from performing any deliveries. If the midwife tested positive for syphilis, she had to undergo treatment and a doctor had to indicate when it was safe for her to perform deliveries again.[65] In 1928 nurse A. E. McDaniel of Tishomingso County reported that "the one who had a positive Wassermann is taking treatment regularly and we hope we can give her a permit before long. She asks about her permit each time she comes in."[66]

Midwives also lost their permits when they delivered pregnant women who had syphilis, unless the women were receiving treatment at the county health department. The state believed that syphilis caused many of the miscarriages of pregnant women.[67] Midwives were responsible for getting their patients to treatment appointments. If a woman refused treatment, the midwife was supposed to deny her service. In Adams County in 1931 nurse Ethel B. Marsh mentioned that "one midwife this month has had her permit revoked for waiting on a case she had been told not to take. This is her first offense and, therefore, her permit is only being temporarily held."[68]

In extreme cases health departments called on police power to force compliance with state rules. In 1931 nurse Josie Strum of Clarke County chose to handle one midwife with extraordinary measures as a warning to all midwives. Strum indicated in her report: "Another midwife was discovered practicing midwifery without a permit, warnings did not seem to do any good so we had her arrested. She was convicted and fined. Now she is very anxious for a permit as well as several others in that same neighborhood."[69]

The Mississippi State Board of Health resorted to prosecution for violation of the rule that a midwife had to be a woman. The state tried to stop black and white men from practicing midwifery. Although health officials did not indicate their motivations, they may have believed that women were easier to regulate or that, except for doctors, men had no place in the birthing room. In 1927 a welfare worker in Jones County advised state nursing supervisor Mary D. Osborne that Joe Hatten, Jr., a young black man, was working as a midwife in the county. "I am told he gets all the business," she explained, "and the women have no business at all, among the colored people." The county health officer called Hatten into his office and informed him he was not to practice any longer. The warning was not effective; in 1933 the welfare worker again contacted Osborne about Hatten's midwifery practice. This time Osborne referred the complaint to Dr. R. N. Whitfield, Director of Vital Statistics at the State Board of Health, for prosecution. The final outcome remains unclear.[70]

In later years the state even used its regulatory power to punish midwives engaged in civil rights activity. A former midwife living in Greenville in the 1960s claimed she lost her permit "because I demonstrated and sat in down at Jackson."[71] In numerous ways, nurses helped the state enforce its rules by implementing policy that limited who could and who could not practice with state approval. Yet, midwives found ways to resist regulations, and no doubt many unregistered midwives practiced midwifery clandestinely.

Midwife Responses to Black and White Public Health Nurses

Historical records, especially government documents, rarely tell us much about the responses of midwives to health professionals. However, the records of the Mississippi State Board of Health contain a wealth of correspondence from midwives, in which they described their health activities and lobbied the board of health. In particular, the death of Mary D. Osborne, the state supervisor of nurses and midwives, prompted a deluge of letters to the newly hired supervisor that hint at how midwives viewed this health official as well as their own work. In addition, midwives used their letters to influence board decisions about which nurses were sent to instruct them, often singling out black nurses for praise.

The Death of Mary D. Osborne

Many of Mississippi's white public health nurses came from outside the South because white Southerners tended to associate nursing with black women's low-status servant work and shied away from the profession. Thus it is not surprising that the white state supervisor of nurses and midwives was from Ohio. Mary D. Osborne (1875–1946), a 1902 graduate of the Akron City Hospital nurses' program, served the state from 1921 until her retirement in 1946. Her administration was responsible for the development of the midwife training program. She had a close, cordial working relationship with Dr. Felix J. Underwood: Osborne ran the public health programs, while Underwood lobbied the politicians for funding.[72]

Osborne was a strict supervisor in her work with nurses and midwives, but most of them apparently appreciated her knowledge and learned from her. In 1943 one midwife, Bessie Ann Swearegan, wrote to thank Osborne for a recent visit to the county: "I learn a lots of thing that you told us that the doctor did not seems to know." Further on she stated: "I love you because you is so kind and taken so much pains to give us good understanding and did not scold us but tried to learn us." The midwife continued her blessings on Osborne: "May God let you live a long time because you is upbuilding to the human race."[73]

Osborne lived only three more years; her death in 1946 prompted an outpouring of similar praise from midwives. They sent their responses to Lucy E. Massey, who replaced Osborne as state supervisor, after Massey sent notification of Osborne's death to the midwife club leaders around the state. Interpreting these replies is complicated because, read at one level, the midwives' eulogies to Osborne present a picture of deferential black women bemoaning the loss of their beloved white leader. Such a reading is strikingly reminiscent of white southern fantasies about slave devotion to the plantation mistress. It is possible, however, that some of the midwives liked or respected Osborne. Others may have written letters of condolence as part of southern etiquette. Still others used Osborne's death as an opportunity to make a favorable impression on their new white supervisor by reflecting on their working relationship to their late "boss."[74]

This collection of midwife letters, whose words are quoted here with the original spelling, is not only a testimony to Osborne but also a testimony of the faithful to their own good works. This correspondence deserves further analysis by historians, especially scholars of the religious culture of rural black women.[75] In these letters, midwives wrote of their own personal sorrow on hearing of Osborne's death, and they usually concluded with a broad message about the meaning of life and death. Midwife Mary Cox of Tunica wrote of the news that it "hurt me to my heart to here it. I could not help but cry. Still I new that she had to die and leave us some day but she was a friend to me since 1923 when set up the midwife club in Tunica." Cox noted that "no fault did you fine of my work" and that Osborne was "trying to teach me the good things of life to live for my self, and the mothers and babys. So sleep and take your rest as I says we all love you but God love you best."[76] Midwife Sarah Crosby of Puckett wrote on behalf of her sister midwives: "We certainly did regret much to hear of the death of Miss Mary Osborne. We have lost our leader." She continued: "We shall ever remember that our dear leader watches us from on high. And as she was devoted to us in life, so is she devoted to us in death. God sustain us under this heavy afflication."[77]

The midwife letters were not simply deferential praise to a dead white leader, but expressions of the nature of their religious faith. The women preached about the inevitability of death and the promise of everlasting life in heaven. Midwife Laura E. Scott began with the often repeated refrain that "our loss is heaven's gain."[78] A midwife from Ruleville wrote to Massey: "I want to say we was all shocked very much when we heard of Miss Osborne's death. When I read your letter the tears ran from my eyes. We all—loved her as our supervisor—we will learn to love you too as well I hope. As we work togather we become more acquainted with each other. I know we must give her up, as we all must go in that same direction, as she went."[79]

Midwives viewed themselves as partners in a complex relationship with public health nurses. When Swearegan wrote again to the board of health in 1946, she indicated that she was sorry to hear of Osborne's death and that

> all the good work she has done is over now. We are looking to you as our Supervisor and all good things that you can do to save the lives of Mothers and Babies. She has fought a good fight and has finish her coarse. We will missed her and have been teach under her instruction for 26 years ever since I been a midwife. It our lost but it Heaven gain. Sleep on Mrs. Osborne, sleep on that Everlasting Sleep. I will be there some day![80]

Midwives believed that God rewarded the faithful in a heaven for black and white believers. Although nurses assisted midwives to improve their work, midwives ultimately answered to a higher power.

BLACK PUBLIC HEALTH NURSES

Among the letters of Mississippi midwives there was frequent praise for the work of the state's six black public health nurses, especially Eliza Farish Pillars (see Figure 8).[81] Midwives went out of their way to inform the board of health how much they enjoyed the work of the black nurses and looked forward to seeing them again. For example, in 1935 a midwife from Claiborne County commented that the midwives in her area were "so thankful for those splendid colored nurses you sent us in June and hope some day they will come again. They made it so plain that even the person that can't read can understand."[82] Leatha Johnson reported on a successful midwife meeting in which "Mrs. Eliza Pillars realy instructed us and we realy enjoyed it."[83] In December 1936, midwife Celia Hall spoke highly of Pillars, who had come to instruct them. Hall stated that "she gave a wonderful lecture. I enjoyed every word she said and it was so much needed what she taught. I think all enjoyed for everyone listened with eager ears. I mean to do better another year than I've ever done before if it is possible."[84]

Eliza Farish Pillars (1891–1970), the first black public health nurse hired by the Mississippi State Board of Health, was well known among midwives for her work around the state. Born in Jackson, Mississippi, Pillars graduated from Hubbard Hospital and Nursing School at Meharry Medical College in the 1910s. She worked for a few years as a hospital staff nurse and then worked for the Mississippi State Board of Health from 1926 to 1945.[85] In 1928 Yazoo County nurse Permelia Harris commented that Pillars demonstrated to a group of midwives "How to Equip the Midwife Bag" and "How to Use the Equipment," noting that it "was greatly appreciated by all the midwives, as well as myself."[86] Pillars also taught hygiene

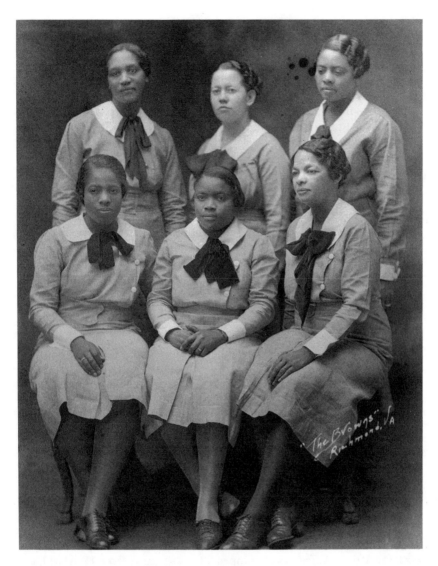

Figure 8. Black public health nurses, Mississippi Board of Health, including Eliza Pillars on the lower right, 1936. Courtesy of the Mississippi Department of Archives and History, Jackson, Mississippi.

classes to young black women studying to become teachers. Some of these young women even trained to became midwives.[87]

In 1945 Pillars retired, according to some accounts, due to weakened eyesight and poor health. However, retired nurse Edna Roberts believed that Osborne forced Pillars to leave because Pillars wanted more rights for black nurses than Osborne was willing to give. For example, in addition to unequal pay, black nurses were given job appointments that differed from those for white nurses. Black nurses in Mississippi were itinerant nurses, which meant that they worked out of the board of health headquarters in Jackson and traveled around the state rather than receive an appointment in one county. No county was willing to hire a black woman as its sole nurse, and only a few counties hired several nurses. Pillars was an activist and, according to Roberts, rightly wanted more respect and better working conditions for black nurses. Her activism was honored by black, and eventually even by white, nurses. In 1951 Pillars became the last recipient of the Mary Mahoney Award from the National Association of Colored Graduate Nurses. A black nurses' organization in Jackson is named in her honor and the Mississippi Nurses' Association entered her in its Nurses' Hall of Fame.[88]

The history of black public health nursing is intricately tied to the state regulation of midwives. Southern state boards of health specifically hired black nurses to assist with training midwives. Generally, health agencies justified white resistance to black health attendants when they stated that black nurses were better suited for work among African Americans than among whites. However, health agency personnel also asserted a position shared by many black leaders, that black nurses were more effective than white nurses in reaching black people because black clients were more likely to trust other black people.[89]

The U.S. Children's Bureau even hired a black female physician, Dr. Ionia Whipper, to assist nurses in southern states to train midwives in the belief that black health professionals were most effective in public health work for African Americans. Whipper, a 1903 graduate from Howard University Medical School, who had worked at Tuskegee Institute in the early 1920s, worked for the Children's Bureau from 1924 to 1929, when the expiration of Sheppard-Towner funds led to her termination. She traveled for the bureau from state to state in the South, training midwives and locating midwives who states had missed in their registration drives. Later, she opened a home for unwed mothers after working at a women's clinic in Washington, D.C.[90]

Occasionally problems developed between midwives and public health nurses, even when both were African Americans. In 1938, nurses Eliza Pillars and Gertrude Perkins apparently criticized a midwife for having incomplete birthing equipment during an inspection. The midwife had left her sterile dressings, used during delivery, at home, and they had scolded her. The midwife appealed to Osborne to talk to the nurses. She asked Osborne to forgive her for forgetting the dressings and explained that the nurses were "not to be blame for it either. It realy was me because those girls realy tells us what we must do. They show us everything you wants us to do." She wanted Osborne to tell the black nurses, one in particular, not to be angry with her. She wrote: "I want you to tell my girl that come to my house dont get all mad at me. I wont do her like that any more. I love those girls."[91] Perhaps the midwife resented the scolding and chose to appeal to a higher authority for help. Alternatively, she may have feared that because of her mistake the black nurses would not return again, so she sought to make amends to their supervisor.

The Public Health Work of Midwives

Even though nurses never treated midwives as their equals, they did frequently note midwife contributions to public health work in black communities.[92] In the early 1930s Underwood observed that midwife supervision, which was "primarily designed to render least harmful to the public health the services of these midwives, has converted them into important allies in the cause of human well-being."[93] Thus, health reform in Mississippi developed out of a dynamic interaction between health professionals and poor women.[94]

Midwives seized on the resources provided by public health nurses in order to assist their communities. They became an important conduit for health education in their childbirth work and elsewhere. They provided health instruction to adults and children through the churches and schools. The activities of midwife Mollie Gilmore of Vicksburg during 1936 and 1937 illustrate the range of midwives' health work and their pride in the accomplishments. Gilmore accompanied a public health nurse in home visits to mothers and encouraged people to go to a local church for typhoid shots. "By my influence," she noted, "Dr. Smith was able to protect 80 people from typhoid fever." Gilmore gave health lectures at church and "prayed to the congregation after service." In the fall of 1936 she "talked to

100 different people on prenatal care, and health and care of the baby. During that time I referred 5 expectant mothers to doctor." In addition, she assisted a doctor with the home deliveries of four white women, and she worked on the annual May Day child health program.[95]

Midwives performed important public health work when they encouraged women to receive prenatal and postnatal care, often bringing them to the health department or mothers' clinics themselves. Retired county health officer Dr. W. E. Riecken, Jr., noted that midwives often accompanied their clients to the county health department for checkups and "frequently assisted in the exam room."[96] Midwives also aided the work of nurses by notifying them when a woman had a baby. In 1931 nurses in Sharkey and Issaquena counties reported that they "have tried to visit more lying-in cases this month but it is hard to know when they are confined. Quite a number of midwives report their cases to us right after delivery and in that way we have come in contact with more mothers during the lying-in period."[97] A 1953 Georgia Department of Health midwife training film, *All My Babies*, illustrated the important role of midwives in promoting preventive medical care for pregnant women, even as it reinforced the idea that midwives were to defer to the wisdom of nurses and doctors.[98]

Midwives saw themselves as important liaisons between poor black women and white health professionals. Midwife Maude Bryant in North Carolina remembered that during one unusually difficult labor she called in a doctor to help the woman. The doctor made a rather cursory examination and stated to the onlookers that nothing was wrong and that "Maude's just scared." As he proceeded to leave, the midwife picked up his bag and walked him outside where she firmly told him the woman was very sick, the delivery was not going along well, and "something must be done, and I want you to go back in there." She eventually convinced him to go back to the woman and take her to a hospital. The cumulative affect of such actions by midwives improved poor women's access to medical services.[99]

Midwives advocated increased health care for the poor from nurses as well as doctors. In one case a midwife made requests of the local public health nurse to tend to a sick woman. In 1939 midwife Estelle W. Christian notified nurse Viola M. Jones that a woman had come to see her at a house where she had just delivered a baby. The middle-aged woman had sores on her arms, legs, and buttocks. The midwife explained to the woman that she could not visit with the new mother or baby because she might infect them. Then the woman told the midwife that the family across the road from her had the same symptoms. The midwife wrote the nurse:

Now could you go out there at once to see about this. I made a lecture on the 4th Sunday in August at a church at Willows, Miss. to the people about their health. . . . I advised them if they had any sores or the least suspicion they were infected with that dreaded disease syphilis to please tell some one before it is too late. So she says she heard me talk that day and when she heard I was in the neighborhood she came to tell me about it. So I advised her to stay at home until I talked with you. So if you could come out here one day I could go to their homes with you.[100]

The nurse was so impressed by the midwife that she sent Osborne a copy of the letter indicating that "this is from one of the midwives who is doing so much to educate her people that I feel real proud of her and I wanted you to see this letter."[101] Although the nurse seems to take credit for the helpful actions of the midwife, this example highlights the way that midwives facilitated public health work.

Midwives assisted with venereal disease control work by encouraging pregnant women and other people in the community to have their blood tested. During the early 1920s, Dr. Roscoe C. Brown and his assistants at the Division of Venereal Disease worked among midwives with the expectation that midwives "will help to spread information regarding venereal diseases not only to expectant mothers but to others and that they will become valuable aids in preventive work."[102] In 1944 several nurses wondered why attendance at a venereal disease clinic suddenly increased until they discovered that "a leader of a midwife club who had received literature on syphilis had made talks at churches, schools and in the homes. This midwife was instrumental in sending in several young girls under sixteen years of age who had infectious syphilis."[103]

As a community leader, midwife endorsement of public health projects contributed to community cooperation. Midwives assisted health department efforts to protect African Americans against typhoid fever and diphtheria. They promoted this preventive work at their midwife club meetings, churches, and schools.[104] In 1931 nurse Ethel B. Marsh of Adams County mentioned that her county sponsored an antidiphtheria campaign among black infants and preschool children. She related that "the midwives in the various sections of the county are assisting by informing parents of the various stations and dates on which toxin-antitoxin will be given."[105] Elsewhere in the state, nurse Nell E. Austin of Forrest County indicated that

the midwives are very helpful in getting the colored people immunized against typhoid fever. At the last midwives meeting they were asked to round up all the children in their neighborhoods and bring them to the health department and have them inoculated against typhoid fever. One midwife was in the office the very next morning with fifty-five children.[106]

Nurse Edna U. Edwards in Pearl River County repeated a similar story when she discovered that two midwives of the Dinkmans Midwife Club had assembled a large crowd for typhoid vaccines by canvassing the neighborhood and notifying people of the time and place.[107] Parents knew and trusted their local midwives and more readily permitted their children to participate in health programs that midwives endorsed.

Mothers and other community members were eager to improve their own health and that of their children. Connie Peak Higdon, a nurse in Copiah County, detected extensive community support for protection against diphtheria, typhoid fever, and smallpox. "The colored mothers are asking for the toxin-antitoxin for their children" to guard against diphtheria, she noted. "In one community almost all the colored people had typhoid vaccine last year and had not been sick since so they came back for more. We vaccinated almost all of them against smallpox."[108] In 1937 a nurse at Massey Island in Leflore County reported that "although everyone was very busy picking cotton, these mothers left the fields long enough to bring the babies to the public health nurse to be protected against diphtheria."[109]

Midwives assisted with official health department programs and national public health campaigns. State health officials learned that midwives ran May Day programs on child health and "participated freely in the yearly Negro Health Week activities."[110] In 1935 a midwife in Smith County noted that at their May Day program "a talk was given about the care of the teeth. A few weeks later the peddler who sells extracts, spices, and tooth paste asked the leader of the midwife club what in the world had caused so many of the people in the community to buy tooth paste."[111]

Midwives also successfully organized their own health clinics and health conferences. In 1928 in Coahoma County six midwife clubs organized preschool children's health conferences.[112] In 1935 midwives offered their homes for health conferences, and one midwife even "had a special examining table built." Another midwife worked up such interest in the physical examinations that "upon arrival the physicians and nurses found a house filled with patients. . . . Two white women, one an antepartum and the other a postpartum case, hearing of the conference were so desirous of this service they asked and were of course permitted to come to the home of this midwife."[113] In 1936 in Monroe County midwife Virginia Thompson reported:

We as midwives decided to do some real health work in the rural district besides the May Day program and continue this work twelve months in the year. So with the cooperation of our churches, schools, communities, 4H Clubs, home demonstration agent, health officials and nurses, we organized a health center in each community where expectant mothers meet once per month for examination and advice.[114]

Midwives asserted their authority as community health leaders and expanded their public health offerings at every opportunity.

Midwives provided valuable information and assistance to government agencies beyond the board of health. In the 1930s they assisted with statewide surveys of the blind for the Mississippi State Commission for the Blind and a survey of the disabled for the Civilian Rehabilitation Division of the Mississippi State Department of Education. They also aided county studies on venereal disease, hookworm, and tuberculosis.[115] Furthermore, midwives aided the efforts of southern states to collect vital statistics. State officials attempted to collect data so the states would be included in the federal registration area, which included those states that collected vital statistics information about births and deaths. It was not until the mid-1930s that all states met the federal requirements for their inclusion.[116] Mississippi and other states required midwives to file birth certificates for each birth they attended, which forced illiterate women to find someone else to fill out the forms. States also wanted all stillbirths recorded in order to learn the full extent of infant deaths.

Midwives were well aware of their health care contributions and saw themselves as part of a great health crusade. A Simpson County midwife wrote to Mary D. Osborne, "yes the sisters is praying the time to hasten so they can meet you again for further instruction. They think it so grand that old as they are they can do this great work to help foster in this great battle field of deficiency."[117] One midwife even contacted the board of health asking for official public recognition of the work performed by midwives. She pointed out that there was a Thanksgiving Day, Christmas Day, Mother's Day, and Father's Day and "it look to me we could have a Midwife Day—i ben on this job sense September 1900 an my work been close to a 1,000, an i am workin in my 81 year."[118]

MODEL BIRTHING ROOM DEMONSTRATIONS

One of the more innovative forms of public health education provided by midwives was the model birthing room demonstration. The model delivery room was similar to other extension work demonstration projects of the

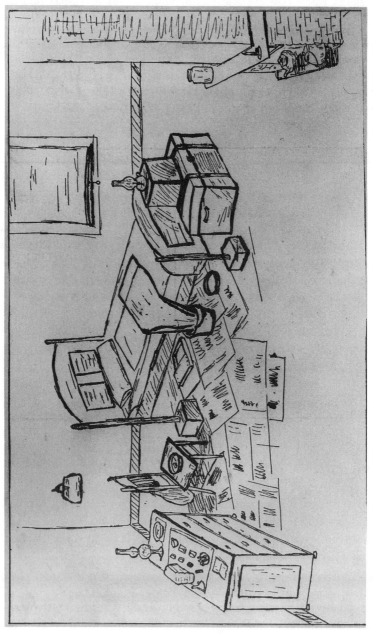

Figure 9. Model delivery room. Courtesy of the Mississippi Department of Archives and History, Jackson, Mississippi.

time in that it operated on the principle of education through first-hand observation. Beginning in the early 1930s the Mississippi State Board of Health required midwives to provide their communities with information about ideal home birthing environments. Twice a year midwives set up a model room in their homes and invited clients and other people in the community to visit. The purpose was to encourage the midwife to demonstrate to the public the correct setup for delivery and to educate future mothers and community members about modern childbirth requirements. The delivery room was supposed to be a neatly organized, clean bedroom, with newspapers spread on the floor and adequate lighting and heating. On the bed was a paper pad with a drip sheet leading into a bucket, no doubt to keep the bed clean in order to reduce the likelihood of postpartum infection by removing discharges (see Figure 9).[119]

It was a clever way to ensure that midwives would be familiar with state regulations, and it also provided publicity about the state health board's work with midwives. A sizable number of midwives complied with the requirement. For example, in 1934 over 1,300 midwives sent in reports of their model delivery rooms. Plantation owners, insurance agents, doctors, teachers, students, mothers, and tenant farmers all attended the demonstrations. It was not uncommon for a midwife to report that she had over a hundred visitors. Black and white, male and female guests examined the room and listened to a description of it by the midwife. Midwives provided paper for people to write down their testimonials or requested that visitors send in their responses to the board of health.[120]

Letters to the board of health attest to the care that midwives put into these demonstrations and illustrate community interest in health education. For example, in 1934 J. M. Boyd, a white registrar and businessman in Louin, indicated that he had inspected the room and equipment of midwife Bertha Smiley and noted that "she is doing a great work among her race to raise the standard of her profession and her work is very commendible. She should be given the very highest rating. I trust your department will continue to give her every help and encouragement possible."[121]

Evaluations seemed to repeat what midwives must have described about the importance of these rooms. White visitors to one model room responded that they "gladly testify that the demonstration was very interesting, sanitary, and modern."[122] Mrs. B. S. Peques of Itta Bena was very impressed with the layout of midwife Matilda Holt Mitchell's room and commented to the board: "I am not overstressing it when I say considering the arrangement of the room, preparation of the bed, the neat and sanitary surroundings it was a fair rival to most hospitals." She continued, "Old ideas and methods have been relegated and replaced by the modern, scientific and streamlined ideas and methods."[123] A doctor who attended this same midwife's room commented that "Aunt" Matilda Holt Mitchell had done an excellent job. He prophesied that "if and when the practice of midwifery conforms to the pattern of this room, in all the cabins and cottages, where negro babies are born, over the south, infant mortality and puerpural sepsis, can and will be largely reduced."[124]

It was clear to black visitors in particular that midwives tried to use what little resources they had available to them to improve the childbirth experiences of poor mothers. In 1941 Mrs. Elliott Thompson visited a model delivery room set up by midwife Lula B. Hudson at Rust College for student teachers. Thompson remarked that "it was a source of inspiration to see what could be accomplished with so little." Mat Jones wrote of the same room that he "enjoyed it because it was the best poor mothers could have when they do not have things they need most."[125] In numerous ways, midwives served changing community needs with a wide range of childbirth and public health care provisions. Furthermore, as women of their communities, they reached far more people than public health nurses ever could.

The Decline of Midwifery

Even though individual nurses commented in their reports on the valuable public health work performed by midwives, ultimately the official policy of the Mississippi State Board of Health remained to eliminate midwives in favor of professional health care. In 1948 nurse supervisor Lucy E. Massey instituted a retirement program, first suggested to her by county nurses, in an effort to accelerate the elimination of midwives.[126] The plan strongly encouraged the retirement of older midwives by informing them and their families that they were too old to renew their permits and then honoring the women with ceremonies, complete with badges stating "Mary D. Osborne Retired Midwife." According to the new policy, "the midwife must promise not to practice and must hand in her permit when she receives the badge."[127] From 1948 on, not only did the state implement this retirement policy but all new midwives had to get a physician to testify that there was a need for their services in the community before they could receive a permit.

The retirement ceremonies probably failed to provide an incentive to leave the practice of midwifery, but they did provide an opportunity for the nurses and people in the community to honor the women. The public health nurse usually held the event at a local church where the midwife "would sit queen for the day."[128] Sometimes people would drop money in the retiring midwife's lap, especially women the midwife had attended. In November 1948 midwives Mollie Merrill and Josephine Franklin were honored in a retirement ceremony at St. John Methodist Church in Forrest County. According to a newspaper report of the event, "the aged pair, clad in white uniforms and caps, and clutching small American flags, sat solemnly in pink and white decorated chairs of honor, placed near the altar." The white county nurse and the black midwife club leader each offered speeches of praise for the women. Those attending sang hymns as the members of the local midwife club led a procession, "robed in white uniforms and caps, and also carrying tiny American flags." Midwives sang, read scripture, offered up prayers, and presented gifts to the retiring midwives.[129]

After 1950 the Mississippi State Board of Health enacted a general policy that discouraged midwives from serving as birth attendants and advocated that midwives only assist women before and after hospital deliveries. In 1951 health officials stated:

> We believe that as soon as possible and as rapidly as possible midwives should be prohibited from delivering any patients either white or colored. . . . We believe that our time and effort is better spent in educating people to use our hospital and medical facilities and in redirecting and retraining midwives to carry out the simple functions for which they are fitted.[130]

Like most health officials, retired nurse supervisor Edna Roberts did not view the end of midwifery as a loss. Although she granted that women might have received less personal contact, she believed that better and more enlightened care through medical science replaced the inferior folk practices of midwives.[131]

Several factors contributed to the decline in the number of Mississippi midwives registered with the state in the post-World War II era. The decreasing numbers were due to state public health policy, but also to such factors as the mechanization of cotton picking, which led to unemployment, and urban migration, which resulted in fewer black midwives living on the surrounding plantations. Furthermore, less women sought midwives when federal initiatives for the construction of hospitals and welfare provisions made it possible for poor southern women to give birth in a hospital. Instead of thousands of registered midwives, by 1966 only 600 midwives had permits in the state, although they still delivered 10,000 to 12,000 babies that year. By 1975 there were only 220 registered midwives who delivered about 1,000 babies. In 1982 the state had a mere 13 registered lay midwives, by which point the state no longer issued permits or held training sessions.[132] The heyday of midwifery was over.

Conclusion

Midwives played an important but overlooked historical role as public health workers for rural African Americans. From 1920 to 1950 African-American midwives broadened their responsibilities for community health care, even as state regulation set limitations on their activities. Ironically, state regulation created an opportunity for midwives, long concerned with the health of their communities, to assist nurses in implementing state health policy. Indeed, black health reform in the rural South depended on the work of women at the bottom of the medical hierarchy — African-American midwives.

6. Sharecroppers and Sorority Women
The Alpha Kappa Alpha Mississippi Health Project

Even with the public health work of black midwives, Mississippi still symbolized the worst aspects of health deprivation and economic oppression in the country. In the midst of the Great Depression, the poverty and ill-health of rural African Americans in the Mississippi Delta caught the attention of a group of black sorority women who concluded it was their duty as middle-class African Americans to serve the black poor. Members of the Alpha Kappa Alpha (AKA) Sorority designed, financed, and carried out the Alpha Kappa Alpha Mississippi Health Project for two to six weeks every summer from 1935 to 1942. Much like black club women during the Progressive Era, middle-class members of AKA attempted to conduct racial uplift work through addressing the social welfare needs of the poor. However, unlike earlier club women, from the very beginning AKA leaders coordinated their private efforts for public health with government officials at the local and national level.

At a time of New Deal promises, AKA leaders shared the rising expectations of African Americans who urged the federal government to implement a second Reconstruction. Black sorority leaders used the AKA Mississippi Health Project to focus federal attention on the destitute conditions of African Americans in the rural South, where the Depression took its heaviest toll. Despite ongoing black migration, this region was still home to most black people in the 1930s.[1]

The history of the AKA Mississippi Health Project typifies the way black health reform straddled the line between social service work and political activity. In order to improve health conditions for sharecroppers in the Mississippi Delta, AKA leaders had to do more than establish clinics. They had to secure the cooperation of the predominantly white federal, state, and county health officials. They also had to overcome resistance from plantation owners who feared the women were little more than "outside agitators" interfering in southern labor relations. In an attempt not to alienate any necessary players, AKA leaders consciously censored criticism of "white power" in their annual reports on the health project. At the same time, they had to reassure black sharecroppers that there was no risk involved in participating in the health clinics. Through the Mississippi Health Project, the sorority engaged in a diplomatic as well as health mission.

The Class Gap: Black Professionals and Black Peasants

Although members of AKA shared a history of racial oppression with those they aided, they did not share similar class positions. Black female students at Howard University in Washington, D.C., founded AKA, the oldest black sorority in the United States, in 1908. AKA recruited black college leaders and academic achievers from historically black colleges and predominantly white colleges across the country. Many of the college sorority members continued their affiliation after graduation. At the time of the health project, the sorority had over 2,000 members in 125 chapters around the country, including both undergraduate and alumnae chapters.[2]

Personal circumstances differed dramatically between the AKA health project volunteers and the black sharecroppers who lived like peasants in the Mississippi Delta. The educational background, urban residence, and moderate economic security of the middle-class sorority women separated them from the sharecroppers who faced harsh living and working conditions. The flat delta, which was settled through levee construction and railroads at the turn of the century, was part of the Mississippi River floodplain in the northwestern part of the state. By 1910 Delta cotton plantations produced prosperity for planters and poverty for sharecroppers, who lived in small cabins with only a few rooms, no plumbing, and an outdoor privy (toilet). Malnutrition was a serious problem because many plantation owners did not want tenants to spend time away from cash crops tending home gardens. Most food, therefore, had to be purchased at the plantation store, which offered only limited items, mostly salt, sugar, grits, cornmeal, molasses, and fatback. Sharecroppers' difficulties were compounded by limited formal education and a political system characterized by such practices as poll taxes and intimidation from an entrenched white elite. Not surprisingly, in the 1930s less than one-half of one percent of black adults ever voted in Mississippi and other Deep South states.[3]

Such distinct class and cultural differences between the AKA women and the Mississippi sharecroppers both motivated and complicated the sorority's health activism. The sorority women viewed themselves as superior to the black poor, yet at least some members felt a keen sense of responsibility for their welfare because "every Negro is a standard bearer for the race."[4] As the first annual report of the health project explained, it was "absolutely the duty of every Negro who has had advantages to go down to these benighted people and administer — personally — to their needs. There cannot possibly be any hope for perceptible elevation of the racial mass otherwise."[5] Their racial uplift goals were intertwined with efforts to secure their middle-class position. As the health report's authors wrote, "there can be no top — if the bottom is not solidly there."[6]

The sorority members were aware that the gap in material resources between the poor and the middle class had created class tensions. As one of the annual health project reports explained:

> perhaps the most tragic aspect of these differences . . . is the gap they have created between the Negro masses who have not yet emerged from the sub-standard mode of life and a Negro minority which has attained a high cultural level. Since this minority believes that it has been stigmatized by the status of the sub-standard masses, and they [the poor] feel completely repudiated by the more fortunate, a keen resentment has developed between the two.[7]

The Mississippi Health Project was an attempt on the part of black middle-class women to bridge that class gap and demonstrate a social conscience toward the difficulties of the black poor.[8]

Ida Louise Jackson and the AKA Summer School for Rural Teachers

AKA's social welfare work in Mississippi began in 1934 with a teacher education program directed by Ida Louise Jackson, the president of the sorority from 1933 to 1937. Jackson (1902-), a native of Mississippi, moved to Oakland, California, in 1918 with her family. Resisting racial barriers, in the mid-1920s she fought successfully to become the first black teacher hired in the Oakland public schools. Jackson was a highly educated woman who earned a bachelor's degree in education in 1922 and a master's degree in 1923 from the University of California at Berkeley, where she helped to start a chapter of AKA. She also did doctoral work at Columbia Teachers College. Jackson followed the advice of her father, who told her to "get an education. That's the one thing that the white man can't take from you."[9]

Jackson launched an education program in Mississippi after she discovered the desperate situation of the black poor in the Delta. In 1933 Jackson attended a fund-raising concert in Oakland by girls from the Saints Industrial and Literary School of Lexington, Mississippi, a religious school headed by Dr. Arenia C. Mallory. Jackson was dismayed at Mallory's descriptions of the bleak conditions in Mississippi. She could not understand why the government did not help and thought it was time that the nation's leaders helped those who could not help themselves. Jackson spoke to Mallory after the concert and developed a plan to donate books to the school. That Christmas Jackson decided to visit her previous home state and was appalled by the extreme poverty and inadequate educational facilities. It seemed to her that the situation had worsened since her childhood. Therefore, in 1934 she garnered AKA support and launched the AKA Summer School for Rural Teachers as a way to improve the quality of education for black children by upgrading local teachers. Jackson selected six teachers to serve as instructors from among the AKA volunteers and paid them from her own pocket, supplemented by funds from the sorority. She publicized the sorority's summer program in Holmes County in the Associated Negro Press and on NBC radio.[10]

Although Jackson initially saw education as the key to improving conditions for southern African Americans, she soon changed her mind and concluded that health conditions had to be improved before educational opportunities would be meaningful. According to Jackson, her opinion changed after traveling around to the plantations and "seeing the homes of the poor people living in the most unsanitary conditions. It was unbelievable."[11] She concluded that malnutrition, decayed teeth, eye problems, and the effects of syphilis and tuberculosis had to be addressed first.[12]

Unlike the attitude of earlier club women who felt that any woman could perform public health work, by the period of the 1930s Jackson felt compelled to garner medical expertise as well as sorority authorization and funding. As head of the sorority, she again approached the sorority membership at the annual convention and argued that AKA should carry out the project on the grounds that it was important for the race. In her message to the membership, Jackson emphasized that "they had to know that we were lucky, that we could have been in that condition."[13] AKA members voted approval of the project, and the sorority provided $1,500 to help cover the costs. Jackson then appointed a committee to organize the health project. The health committee, composed of doctors, nurses, and laywomen, circulated a questionnaire to all AKA members and, after receiving the responses, decided the project should begin with a focus on children's health.

Southern children were an appropriate focus, the committee noted, because children were the hope of the future and the South was the most impoverished region. On the recommendation of Jackson's friend and AKA founder Norma Boyd, Jackson asked sorority member Dr. Dorothy Boulding Ferebee to join the project as medical director.[14]

Health Missionaries: Dr. Dorothy Boulding Ferebee and the AKA Volunteers

Dr. Dorothy Boulding Ferebee (1898–1980) directed the work of the Mississippi Health Project on top of her job at Howard University, her private practice, and raising her young twins. Born in Virginia, Ferebee grew up in Boston. She earned degrees at Simmons College in 1920 and Tufts Medical College in 1924. At Tufts she was one of five women in a class of 137 medical students. According to Ferebee, "we women were always the last to get assignments in amphitheaters and clinics. And I? I was the last of the last because not only was I a woman, but a Negro, too."[15] Despite these obstacles, Ferebee graduated in the top five of her class and, after repeated rejections by white hospitals, secured an internship in Washington, D.C., at Freedmen's Hospital. Following her internship, Howard University hired her in 1927 as an instructor of obstetrics at the medical school. She also gained experience lobbying public officials during her effort to establish a social settlement in Washington, D.C., in 1929 (see Figure 10).[16]

Ferebee selected health project volunteers on the basis of previous relevant experience. She chose twelve AKA members to participate in the Mississippi Health Project that first summer, including one doctor, two nurses, and several teachers and social workers. For some women it was difficult to be away from their jobs for so long, and the doctor, Zenobia Gilpin, had to withdraw at the last moment because of the demands of her practice. AKA workers were not paid, but AKA used membership dues to reimburse the volunteers for their expenses in laundry and room and board.[17]

Probably no one was better qualified than public health nurse Mary E. Williams. Williams, a graduate of Hampton Institute and Richmond Hospital Nurses Training School, knew Ferebee from her days in Virginia. Williams worked as a school nurse for Henrico County, Virginia, during World War I, and in 1922 she was hired for the Tuskegee Movable School in Alabama. Later that same year she became head of the newly founded

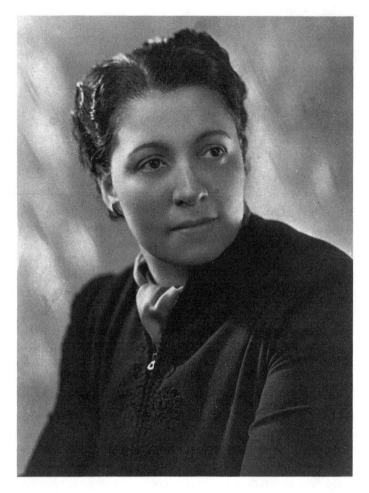

Figure 10. Dr. Dorothy Boulding Ferebee. Courtesy of the Bethune Museum and Archives, Washington, D.C.

Tuskegee Institute Health Center, which provided free health care to three-fourths of the residents of Macon County, Alabama. In 1924 Williams received a scholarship from the American Child Hygiene Association, and she studied public health for a short time at Simmons College in Boston. In the 1930s she won a scholarship from the Rosenwald Fund to take course-work at Harvard University School of Public Health. Williams, who was very active in social service work, organized a settlement house in New Orleans in 1927, attended National Negro Health Week planning meetings in Washington, D.C., and worked with projects of the Tuskegee Woman's Club.[18]

It was Williams, with her work experience in the rural South, who suggested that Ferebee contact the county health officer in Holmes County and the local doctors in order to avoid any misunderstandings. Williams urged Ferebee to follow her advice, stating: "I know the south better than you or Zenobia do, especially the FAR south." She reminded Ferebee that it would be difficult to run clinics "unless the doctors down this part of the south KNOW that you are NOT going to start something to take their practice away from them. . . . You are NOT going to succeed unless you can be very diplomatic."[19]

DELTA CLINICS AND CONFLICT

The sorority volunteers encountered many difficulties in carrying out their plans for the health project, yet they demonstrated resiliency and creativity in the face of white resistance. Because the volunteers lived across the nation, from New York to Ohio to California, they decided to meet at Ferebee's home in Washington, D.C., and take the train to Mississippi together. When a white railway agent refused to sell train tickets to Ferebee, due to the limited seating for African Americans in segregated trains, the sorority women decided to borrow cars and drive there. They drove to Mississippi despite the load of medical supplies they had to transport and the travel difficulties African Americans faced during segregation. As Ferebee recalled, it was "a 2,000 mile run over unknown roads, many without restroom facilities, or over night accommodations, or even gas stations willing to serve black travellers."[20]

The AKA participants faced more difficulties upon reaching Mississippi. They set up their headquarters at the Saints Industrial and Literary School in Holmes County, where they could obtain food and lodging. The plan was to hold the health clinics from 9:00 A.M. to 4:00 P.M. six days per week for six weeks at the Saints School, with lectures for adults in the evening. The clinic opened as planned in a boys' dormitory at the school, but after their first few days of clinic operation the attendance was very low. The women tried to find out why and learned that white plantation owners, wary of "outside agitators," refused to allow "their" sharecroppers to leave the plantations and attend the clinics. According to Jackson, plantation owners "did not want their people to leave the land for fear they might not come home."[21] Undaunted, the AKA women agreed among themselves that they had not come all this way for nothing. According to Ferebee, the

AKA volunteers concluded, "Well, if they can't come to us, we'll go to them."[22] The women turned their cars, which they were forced to bring in the first place, into mobile health clinics and drove out to each plantation. The result was that the health project reached far more people than any centralized clinic ever would have.[23]

The project also saw conflict beyond that caused by white planters. Tensions developed among the volunteers and Arenia Mallory. Several of the volunteers described Mallory as hard to work with and too eager to take credit for the whole project. Even before heading for Mississippi, Jackson had warned Ferebee about possible problems and that "Miss Mallory is *very* sensitive about 'not belonging' — I think you know what I mean for we Sorors can make other people feel they had no right to be born if we so desire." After the summer project, Williams described Mallory as a deceitful, jealous, dangerous person who should be avoided at all costs. Although the project was located in Holmes County in the first and last years, from 1936 to 1941 AKA ran the project in neighboring Bolivar County. Ferebee was relieved not to return to Holmes County.[24]

In Bolivar County, the all-black town of Mound Bayou provided comfortable accommodations and served as headquarters for the health project. Initially AKA leaders had considered taking the program to other states with similar conditions, such as Florida, Louisiana, and Alabama, but Dr. Martha Elliot, Assistant Chief of the U.S. Children's Bureau, urged Ferebee to remain in Mississippi where the groundwork had been laid. Mound Bayou, with a population of about 800, was also an attraction for the health project because of the support of most residents. The mayor helped the sorority get permission from the county school board to hold health clinics in black schools, and he widely advertised the project so that landowners would be less resistant to the idea.[25]

Bolivar County also proved to be a good choice because the sorority volunteers received valuable assistance from the white county health officer, Dr. Rosier D. Dedwylder. Dedwylder (1882–1948) was born in Alabama and earned his medical degree from the University of Alabama. In 1920 he became the full-time county health officer in Bolivar County. He carried out that job for 28 years until his death. Jackson remembered Dedwylder as surprisingly cooperative. She and Ferebee observed Dedwylder's interactions with people in the county and were impressed by his efforts on behalf of the black sharecroppers. He knew how to convince the landowners to cooperate by insisting that the health project was in their interest because healthier workers meant the planters made more money. With a budget of only twenty-five cents per person, at a time when white counties in the state spent one dollar per person, Dedwylder knew that AKA helped him do his job. AKA acknowledged his support in the 1941 annual health report and described him as a man "whose whole-hearted enthusiasm and cooperation are among the outstanding highlights of our six years service."[26]

The conditions within which the AKA women worked in the Delta were not ideal, even though critics among sorority members envisioned the health project as merely an AKA-funded vacation for a few. Ferebee remarked, "Those at home who thought we were down in Mississippi having a big time should have been there to see what difficulties we experienced."[27] Jackson even reported to the sorority members after the first year, "If anyone Soror is desirous of doing missionary work — 'See America First' before going to Africa."[28] The women found that the most accessible places to hold clinics were in small black churches, often the only black-controlled institution. Jackson remembered that "many of these churches served also as the only school in the area. At other times we set up our equipment under the trees. On one occasion we had to use the porch of a plantation owner's house (under close supervision of the owner)."[29] Jackson remembered that the plantation owners were extremely suspicious. "It was so sad to see these white owners standing around trying to hear what was going on," she explained. "When the medical team did not want them to know what was happening, all they had to do was speak in the language of the profession."[30]

Despite the dusty country roads and inadequate facilities, the sorority women ran their clinics professionally, with as much order and efficiency as possible. They set up clinic tables with crisp, white linen and put on matching white uniforms in order to "give an air of healthfulness and cleanliness." Teachers, such as Marion Carter from St. Louis, Missouri, and nurses, such as Mary E. Williams from Tuskegee Institute, took patients' health histories and prepared children for immunizations, while Ferebee gave the injections.[31]

As was typical of public health work during the 1930s, the AKA health project included venereal disease control work. From the start, Jackson had felt such work was a necessary component of the project in the Delta because, as she wrote to Ferebee, "that section is rank with it."[32] The sorority provided Wassermann tests for everyone over twelve, especially pregnant women. The organizers also contacted the United States Public Health Service (USPHS) for educational posters and publications on venereal disease, and Ferebee kept Dr. Raymond Vonderlehr of the Venereal Disease Division informed of the success of their work.[33]

SHARECROPPERS' HEALING TRADITIONS AND REACTIONS TO CLINICS

Out in the Mississippi Delta, AKA professionals encountered folk healers and folk medicine that sometimes shocked them, but they tried to understand them within the context of economic deprivation and political oppression. The AKA health workers regarded as "superstitious" practices such as charms worn around children's necks, perhaps to make teething easier, and an eighteen-month-old baby boy who wore his hair in plaits because his mother was afraid that in cutting his hair she would "cut" his speech.[34] Dr. Edna Griffin of California, who assisted with the health project in 1942, recalled that her "scissors were as busy cutting away conjure bags and moles' feet from the charm strings on the necks of children and grownups as they were cutting bandages."[35] Even if the volunteers did not understand the cultural healing traditions of rural people, such observations only further politicized the sorority women into advocating modern health care for poor black people.

It did not take long for the sorority volunteers to realize that it was the support of midwives, along with ministers, that guaranteed sharecropper attendance at the health clinics. AKA workers met with local midwives, who were at the center of the traditional healing networks in Holmes and Bolivar counties, both of which had populations that were three-fourths African American. In 1935 in Holmes County there were only 77 registered midwives for a population of approximately 24,000 African Americans. In Bolivar County there were 113 registered midwives for some 50,000 African Americans. It is likely that there were more midwives who had not registered with the state, but there were still more midwives than doctors. Bolivar, for example, had only 33 doctors, two of whom were black.[36] Midwives took on an advocacy role for their communities. They provided the AKA health workers with meals and "horrible tales" about the slave-like living conditions of sharecroppers.[37]

It is difficult to uncover the reactions of the black sharecroppers to these health clinics, but given their own healing traditions they most likely felt a mixture of hesitancy and curiosity. The episodic nature of the sorority women's involvement first in Holmes County, then in Bolivar County, no doubt hindered the development of trust, which was well established with the midwives.[38] Perhaps most importantly, the sharecroppers feared the reactions of plantation owners to their interactions with the sorority women. In addition, a few sharecroppers may have been unfamiliar with methods of modern medicine and reluctant to seek out services for themselves, and especially for their children, that appeared to be painful. This report from a sorority volunteer in 1936 gives an indication of the apprehension with which sharecroppers arrived at AKA clinics for children's immunizations:

> The psychology of fear is an interesting thing. Hundreds of parents were in almost total ignorance of the methods and results of the treatment, but for some reason were mortally afraid that "sticking needles in the child's arm would hurt." Easily communicating this fear to their children, they were brought to the clinic so wrought up and hysterical that the touch of a warm soapy cotton applicator made them scream and cry.[39]

It seems reasonable to assume that being poked by a needle would hurt. What is most noteworthy is that despite everything, sharecroppers actually came to the clinics in search of health care.

AKA reports indicate that the sorority women tried creative approaches to persuade the sharecroppers to attend the clinics. Knowing that sharecroppers were wary of outsiders, explained AKA volunteer Ella Payne Moran, clinic staff went to local church services, where they advertised their clinics and attempted to allay fears about white retaliation for clinic participation.[40] The sorority women also emphasized that their clinics were projects by black women health workers for black sharecroppers, in the hope that this fact would encourage participation. Aware of the illiteracy of much of the rural population, the volunteers used visual materials and lined up colorful posters to attract attention and explain the health messages. They also encouraged attendance by providing gifts for the children, including toothbrushes and clothing. In 1939 they gave nutrition lectures and introduced new food items by offering free meals at the end of the day when people were most hungry.[41] Ferebee remembered that "thousands of tenant families came at first timidly as many had never seen a doctor or a nurse. But soon they came in droves."[42] These various strategies helped the health project reach thousands of children and adults.

The Impact of the Mississippi Health Project

The impact of the health project on the black sharecroppers of Mississippi must be analyzed in terms of both the health services brought by the clinics and the changes the project left behind. The AKA clinics supplied physical examinations, vaccinations, nutrition and personal hygiene information, clothing, food items, and treatments for malaria and venereal disease. Dr. Mary C. Wright (Thompson) of Boston provided dental services, including instruction in dental hygiene, and extracted as many as 60 unhealthy teeth per day.[43] The health workers attended to 150 to 300 people each day at the clinics, for a total clinic attendance each summer of from 2,500 to over 4,000 people. The effect on the health of children was perhaps most significant: AKA health staff provided well over 15,000 children with immunization against smallpox and diphtheria.[44]

The health project made a difference well beyond the clinic work. AKA encouraged the people of Mound Bayou in their pursuit of a hospital and urged a local fraternal organization in the town, Sir Knights and Daughters of Tabor, to open one in Mound Bayou instead of following their plans for a new office building. The Taborian Hospital, which opened in 1942 as the county's first black hospital, cost $100,000 and was funded mostly by local black residents and fraternal members. Ida Jackson remembered that, ironically, the man appointed as chief surgeon of Taborian Hospital, Dr. Theodore Howard, had been the one black doctor who did not cooperate with the AKA project because he feared that it was interfering with his private practice.[45] The sorority women also organized several meetings on race relations with white Methodist women in the county, with the result that some of them opened a recreation hall for African American boys run by a black social worker.[46]

Furthermore, the sorority women believed that their mere presence as black professionals offered hope to helpless sharecroppers. Dr. Edna Griffin believed that the reason white people did not readily welcome the presence of the sorority was that "it created a restless yearning among the younger colored people — prompted them to migrate from the Delta to more promising parts of the country."[47] According to the sorority's health report, one sharecropper told the AKA women: "When we heard about youall coming, we just ran outside and thanked God. We been praying for someone to be sent in His name to speak for his poor laboring people."[48] Sorority volunteers saw themselves as "saviors" of the poor who

> flounder in the quagmire of poverty, ignorance and abject squalor. . . . Truly they are, for the most part, a saddened, defeated, submissive lot. Illiterate, helpless, they present an apathetic picture as they start from fields and doorways with expressions at once stupid, vacant and void of hope.[49]

Such sentiments illustrated that even if the sorority volunteers avoided victim-blaming, they still viewed the sharecroppers solely as victims who they were there to rescue.

Perhaps the greatest impact of the Mississippi Health Project was on the more than forty AKA members who volunteered over the years. According to the 1937 annual report, "each worker emerged from the field of service with a deeper insight and a richer understanding of the life, the needs, and the outlook of the agrarian worker of the South."[50] Volunteer Ruth A. Scott described her first day with the health clinic in 1940 as "nothing short of staggering" as she saw the hundreds of people lined up outside the clinic door awaiting the arrival of the sorority women.[51] The annual reports indicated that the women developed a critique of the southern economic system in their analysis of how to improve health conditions, and they believed that real change required altering the entire living and working environment of the sharecroppers.[52] In 1941 Ferebee, who by then was president of AKA, reported that "the Health Project has revealed many significant findings, but none more important than the fact the standard of health is indissolubly linked to all the socio-economic factors of living."[53] The AKA members saw first-hand those factors, especially the poverty, that hindered the lives of sharecroppers.

Their analysis of the root causes of poor health had an effect on both the programs of the clinics and the direction of future AKA projects. Ferebee reported in a 1941 CBS radio broadcast that the desperate situation of the Depression had motivated the sorority women to take action on behalf of the poor:

> Recognizing the distressing problems of the masses of our people, especially at the lowest economic levels, and recognizing the fact that health is one of the primary needs of all underprivileged people, we set out to offer something beyond an academic discussion of the deplorable conditions of this group.[54]

Over the years AKA volunteers tried to address topics that related to socioeconomic conditions that they could help change, such as diet, lavatory facilities, screens on windows, and recreational facilities. The approach of the health project became a combination of clinical operation, health education, and research on socioeconomic conditions.

Public Policy and the AKA Sorority

Even though the sorority ended the Mississippi Health Project in 1942, after investing $20,000, the sorority's health work did not end. The program came to a halt because World War II gas rationing restricted travel. Furthermore, according to Jackson, the project stopped because she could not help organize it anymore and the sorority chose to invest most of its money in war bonds. Instead, AKA encouraged each of its chapters around the country to develop a health committee that would work with local residents and voluntary agencies to increase black people's access to existing health services. Then in 1945 the sorority opened a National Health Office in New York City under Estelle Massey Riddle (Osborne), a professor of nursing education at New York University, in order to coordinate the work of this nationwide network of local AKA health committees.[55]

At a time when the New Deal expanded federal responsibility for the welfare of citizens, AKA leaders turned to government officials to provide endorsements and funding to the health project. Jackson and Ferebee tried to turn AKA's limited voluntary effort into a permanent government-run program. From the very beginning, AKA leaders had informed federal government officials of the progress of the health project. Dr. Roscoe C. Brown of the Office of Negro Health Work at the USPHS endorsed the project and supported the choice of Holmes County because, he noted, it was "one of the active cooperating counties in our National Negro Health Movement."[56] U.S. Surgeon General Hugh Cumming offered the project high praise. AKA approached Dr. Martha Eliot of the U.S. Children's Bureau, Secretary of Labor Frances Perkins, and Alfred E. Smith of the Works Progress Administration for funding for the Mississippi Health Project from federal relief programs and the Social Security Act. Through these contacts Ferebee was able to get a few black nurses and clerks employed through Works Progress Administration funds to assist with the project. Ferebee and Jackson also contacted officials at the Mississippi State Board of Health, including Dr. Felix Underwood and Mary D. Osborne. Finally, they received the endorsement of Mississippi Senator Pat Harrison and Representative Will Whittington.[57]

AKA efforts to gain federal support even reached into the White House, where, on behalf of their sorority, Jackson and Ferebee criticized the New Deal for its failure to reach African Americans. In late 1935 Eleanor Roosevelt invited Jackson and Ferebee to meet with her at the White House to discuss the first summer's health work as well as the problems that black women faced.[58] Roosevelt had read of their project and expressed an interest in it. The AKA leaders hoped her support would aid them in securing financial assistance for the health project. Jackson reported of the meeting:

> First of all, we felt safe in saying that in spite of Federal provisions for relief, this relief program was not reaching the rural Negro. Secondly, if the Negro is to profit by the measures introduced by this Administration, it meant that Negroes would have to be given supervisory and other places of responsibility with "Federal Protection."[59]

Jackson indicated that Roosevelt responded with the suggestion that "possibly our Health Project might become a Federal Project with AKA Supervision — with the proviso that we could find trained persons on relief who could operate or conduct the Project."[60]

The sorority women tried to shape government policy through their demonstration program. The annual reports of the Mississippi Health Project continually referred to the program as a model to be emulated by the government, as merely a demonstration of the possibilities for reaching those people often missed by relief programs. The 1937 health report observed that "certainly a limited project in a single Southern State could not pretend to have quantitative value." Yet "the final achievement of the Mississippi Health Project will be realized only when Federal, State, or County governments adopt the fundamental principles of its technique and expand this service to large-scale proportions."[61]

Although AKA leaders tried to convince the federal government to take over the work, by and large their requests went unheeded. Jackson had felt optimistic about their efforts and that they had put black health conditions "clearly before the public and it was just a matter of time when the national government would enter the field of medical care."[62] Yet, other than endorsements, the federal government offered little more than surplus food items and a few WPA workers to the sorority.

Support at the state level also proved to be disappointing. Frustrated with Mississippi's failure to provide rural African Americans with access to public health facilities, Jackson and Ferebee tried to arrange a meeting with executive officer Underwood, but he refused. In 1943 Jackson appealed to Eliot at the U.S. Children's Bureau for assistance and stated that the sorority wanted to move the project to other states but lacked sufficient funding and did not want to leave Mississippi until changes had been made. "I believe that resources exist," explained Jackson to Eliot, but she did not know where to turn. Eliot's office indicated that one source was Title V of the Social Security Act. The Children's Bureau administered federal grants from Title V to states for maternal and child health work. An employee at the Children's Bureau noted to Eliot that each year Mississippi failed to spend all the funds to which it had access. Yet states had to provide matching funds to receive federal dollars and Underwood resisted offering state resources for a health program he did not control.[63]

Finally, the sorority attempted to shape public policy through the AKA Non-Partisan Council on Public Affairs, established in 1938. While organizations like the National Association for the Advancement of Colored People (NAACP) fought for civil rights through legal strategies in the courts, AKA turned to congressional lobbying. The Council, headed by soror Norma Boyd, was guided by the words of nineteenth-century black reformer Frederick Douglass, who argued: "Power concedes nothing without a demand." The Council, which grew directly out of AKA's public health work, lobbied Congress and government departments in order to promote antidiscrimination legislation and ensure that the federal government responded to the social welfare needs of all Americans. As AKA health volunteer Portia Nickens argued, the sorority needed to work toward both long-term legislative solutions and immediate survival needs. "One phase of the work cannot gain results without the other," she explained.[64] The Council continued for ten years until 1948 when AKA joined with six sororities and fraternities to form the American Council on Human Rights, a similar lobbying group.[65]

BLACK WOMEN AND THE FEDERAL GOVERNMENT

AKA also joined a coalition of black women's organizations to promote black women's rights and shape federal policy. Through the National Council of Negro Women, founded in 1935, black women collectively articulated their desire for a greater role in the nation's leadership.[66] In 1938 AKA participated in a national conference on federal welfare programs organized by Mary McLeod Bethune, president of the National Council of Negro Women. Bethune, the highest-ranking member of Roosevelt's Black Cabinet, was head of the Office of Minority Affairs of the National Youth Administration from 1936 to 1944.[67] Dorothy Ferebee, Bethune's personal physician, represented the AKA on the Council's health committee, and in 1949 she became the second president of the Council.[68]

Historians have paid little attention to black women's attempts to influence the federal government, except for minor interest in Mary McLeod Bethune. Susan Ware's pathbreaking work on women in the New Deal did not even examine Bethune, on the erroneous conclusion that she represented African Americans and not women, as if black women had no gendered interests.[69] Although Bethune was the only black woman to head an office, by the 1930s there were other black women within the federal government, including social worker Vinita Lewis. Lewis worked as a black child welfare specialist at the U.S. Children's Bureau from 1936 to 1945, hired with funding from the Social Security Act.[70]

The National Council of Negro Women challenged federal government officials on their failure to hire more than a few token black women in government positions, especially given that departments hired many white women during the New Deal. As early as 1925 black women leaders, such as Hallie Q. Brown, had appealed for a greater role for black women in the administration of federal government programs, but with little success.[71] In 1938 Bethune organized a conference of the National Council of Negro Women on "The Participation of Negro Women and Children in Federal Programs" in Washington, D.C.[72] Sixty-five black women leaders attended, including Mary Church Terrell, Lugenia Burns Hope, Arenia C. Mallory, Mary E. Williams, and Dr. Dorothy Boulding Ferebee.[73]

Integration was the theme of the conference. Bethune divided the conference into two parts, the first to discuss the issues among the women themselves, and the second to present their recommendations at the White House to Eleanor Roosevelt and federal department administrators, such as Mary Anderson of the U.S. Women's Bureau and Katharine Lenroot of the U.S. Children's Bureau.[74] The conference members, through the resolutions committee, reported their conclusions:

> Our deliberations have indicated that Negro women and children do not participate in Federal Welfare programs to any extent in proportion to their need. It is our advised opinion that this condition is the direct result of our virtual exclusion from the administrative policy forming offices of various Federal department bureaus set up for the administration and execution of the programs for women and children.[75]

The resolutions decried black women's limited access to federal relief programs and challenged the exclusion of agricultural and domestic workers, over half of all black workers, from social security benefits.[76]

The thrust of their argument was that black women's interests would not be represented in health and welfare policy until black women themselves had the opportunity to construct and administer federal policy. The women criticized the government for sex and race discrimination, stating that "it is impossible for any other than a Negro female representative to understand and appreciate the problems of the unemployed Negro woman."[77] Bethune captured the spirit of the conference when she declared that "the day has come now, not tomorrow, but the day has come *now* for us, as Negro women, to be counted among the women of this country who are making the plans and administering the program to the people of America."[78]

The response of the department heads and Eleanor Roosevelt was basically defensive. Roosevelt, although conceding that black women needed more representation, still maintained that not everyone could be included in every department. Mary Anderson and Katharine Lenroot argued that they had a few black women on their staffs, ignoring the fact that they did not hold positions of authority. It is unclear whether real changes occurred in departmental hires because of this conference, yet such a meeting demonstrated that, through their national organizations, middle-class black women struggled to shape the New Deal.

Conclusion

From the very beginning, AKA leaders felt they were making history and widely publicized the accomplishments of their health project. They sent copies of reports on their health project to other organizations in the hope that they would follow suit.[79] One AKA member remarked to Ferebee that black fraternities showed a great deal of interest in the work of AKA. She reported: "Some of the Alpha men said, it was too bad that the men hadn't thought of such a project. I told them the field was very large and we could not stop them."[80] The sorority was proud of its accomplishments and used the mass media to advertise its work. Many journals, including *Survey Graphic*, *Reader's Digest*, and *National Negro Health News*, carried stories about the health project, and, one summer, *Time*'s newsreel division made a motion picture of the staff working in the health clinics.[81] Ferebee gave public lectures about the Delta clinics and even made a CBS radio broadcast.[82] One AKA volunteer nurse, Bessie E. Cobbs from Freedmen's Hospital in Washington, D. C., publicized the project among the nation's nurses in an article she wrote for the *American Journal of Nursing*.[83] The Mississippi Health Project brought national recognition to the sorority and Ferebee.[84]

The project epitomized black women's volunteer health organizing, which had originated among club women at the turn of the century. It also illustrated the ongoing lobbying efforts of African Americans to convince the government to take responsibility for all people's health. It was a small-scale example of the private initiatives carried out by African Americans on behalf of dispossessed individuals across the nation during the first half of the twentieth century. By mid-century members of the black middle-class placed their hopes for improved health conditions on a new reconstructed South and a new federal commitment to the nation's health. Nevertheless, state-level administration of federally funded programs meant that African Americans did not receive an equal share of the benefits of relief.[85]

Finally, black health activists in the era of segregation had to cultivate diplomatic skills to secure their personal safety and circumvent white resistance to social change. Although the annual AKA health reports never explicitly stated that AKA regarded its health work as "civil rights" activity, that is an appropriate description. AKA leaders never spelled out their intentions in official records because they regularly submitted their reports to government health authorities. As Ida Jackson explained, they had to be careful about what they wrote because they were fearful that antagonizing "white power" would be counterproductive to helping sharecroppers.[86] In retrospect both Jackson and Ferebee felt thankful that no violence against the AKA women ever resulted.

The white planters of the Mississippi Delta certainly feared that the sorority women were conducting civil rights activity — they kept watch on the women at the clinics. According to Ferebee, they employed " 'riders' with guns in their belts and whipping prods in their boots; riders who weaved their horses incessantly, close to the clinics, straining their ears to hear what the staff interviewers were asking of the sharecroppers."[87] In later years she recalled that the project was "labelled by those racist Mississippians, as a program organized by meddlesome, communist black women, coming into their Delta to stir up trouble and to incite tenant farmers."[88] Planters' fears were not entirely unfounded: AKA sorority volunteers were but the advance guard of a future army of activists who would seek to transform the South in the coming years.

Conclusion

In the first half of the twentieth century African Americans created their own solutions to black health problems. At least two major themes emerge in this investigation of how they carried out their work: the ongoing black struggle for federal support and the persistence of black women's organizing efforts.

First, black health activism developed in response to diminishing rights in an era when the state assumed ever greater responsibility for social welfare needs. It is in this context that black professionals and community leaders positioned themselves as "ambassadors" for black America in their struggle for federal attention to black needs. They lobbied the state to ensure black access to increasing government provisions, as it became apparent that private organizing efforts to improve black health were not enough.

Early in this century social welfare activists created new federal health and welfare policies, but the benefits of these policies remained out of reach for most black people because federal officials empowered local white authorities to administer programs. It was extremely difficult for public initiatives to reach African Americans when their interests were not protected, as indicated by the general failure of New Deal programs to assist black Southerners.[1] Given all this, even limited access to federal funds made a difference to black people. For example, the Tuskegee Movable School hired its home demonstration agent with funds from the Smith-Lever Act and its public health nurse with funds from the Sheppard-Towner Act, while the Social Security Act enabled the Mississippi State Board of Health to hire several black nurses.

Second, despite the fact that male leaders like Booker T. Washington and Dr. Roscoe C. Brown received credit for creating a black health movement, laywomen and female health professionals were the ones who pioneered grassroots health organizing. Whether as volunteers or paid workers, black women were the vital links between health initiatives and poor African Americans. They were integral to the implementation of black health programs at the local level, and they sustained black communities in the face of institutionalized racial discrimination and government neglect. Whether one examines the promotion of National Negro Health Week or the public health work of midwives, nurses, teachers, home demonstration agents, and club and sorority members, black women were at the heart of health reform.

Furthermore, health reform was a cornerstone of early black civil rights activity. As the history of black women's health activism demonstrates, from 1890 to 1950 black social welfare activity was indistinguishable from racial uplift work. In an era of legalized segregation, health improvement was necessarily tied to the struggle for social change. Focusing on health issues permitted black women an authoritative voice in the realm of political organizing.[2] They exploited the identification of health needs with the domestic realm in order to take on very public roles and engage in a little-recognized form of civil rights work.

After 1950, social welfare issues continued to be a major focus of black women's activism. More studies are needed on the ways in which concerns over health and housing were as integral to the agenda of the modern civil rights movement as voting rights. Housing, for example, which had been a public health topic for female reformers since at least the Progressive Era, was both a social welfare concern and civil rights issue in the late 1940s and 1950s.[3] After World War II, a "medical" civil rights movement emerged, in which activists pushed for the integration of hospitals, medical and nursing schools, and medical and nursing associations. For example, in 1951 the National Association of Colored Graduate Nurses disbanded because black nurses were finally able to join the formerly white American Nurses Association. However, a mere two decades later, ongoing racism led to the establishment of the National Black Nurses' Association.[4]

Racial politics and government indifference to the plight of African Americans continues to have a major impact on the development of American health policies. Ideas about racial differences and black inferiority still influence explanations for black/white health disparities, with the modern version targeting "lifestyle choices" as the cause of high black morbidity and mortality rates. Thus the fact that black infant mortality rates are still twice as high and black maternal mortality rates three times as high as those for whites is attributed to factors like alcohol and drug use and general indifference to prenatal care, rather than to an unhealthy environment, little access to health care, racial oppression, and poverty.[5]

As the 1980s war on welfare, civil rights, and feminism began to dismantle the gains of the social movements of the 1960s, a self-consciously black *women's* health movement emerged. This movement marked a shift from black women organizing for their communities to organizing for themselves. The contemporary black women's health movement asserts that poverty and racism, as well as sexism and homophobia, have contributed to the poor health status of African Americans.[6] The National Black Women's Health Project, with headquarters in Atlanta, Georgia, has spearheaded the movement. In 1983 the organization, along with the National Women's Health Network, sponsored the First National Conference on Black Women's Health Issues at Spelman College. Organizers expected 500 black women to attend; instead nearly 2,000 showed up.[7] The National Black Women's Health Project has continued to grow through national conferences and the development of over 100 local chapters across the country.

Finally, the nation's failure to address ongoing health problems in black communities has required the continuation of volunteer efforts and has even led to the revival of National Negro Health Week, renamed National Black Health Week in the 1990s. Given the history of black health reform, it is no coincidence that black female health professionals and a laywoman are the major organizers of this effort. In 1991 Rena Hawes, a health sciences librarian at Howard University, discovered a 1939 issue of *National Negro Health News*, where she learned about the earlier Negro Health Week activity. She decided to renew the black health week campaign and create an annual health education program for local black elementary school children. Meanwhile Dr. Anita L. Jackson and Dr. Lesa Walden of Vital Signs, a nonprofit entity committed to preventive medicine, launched an effort to revive black health week nationwide. In 1992 they helped organize a lecture series on black health at the Smithsonian Institution to commemorate National Black Health Week in honor of Booker T. Washington. They have since convinced the National Medical Association to help them lobby Congress to designate April as African American health month.[8]

The health care arena continues to be a site for social change and political activism as the nation grapples with how to meet the health needs of millions of underserved and uninsured Americans. Whose interests will be protected and whose will be sacrificed if the health care system is reorganized or if the existing system is maintained? It is clear that health care continues to be both a private need and a public concern, enmeshed in the politics of the day.

Notes

Introduction

1. Charles Payne, "Men Led, But Women Organized: Movement Participation of Women in the Mississippi Delta," in *Women in the Civil Rights Movement*, ed. Vicki L. Crawford, Jacqueline Anne Rouse, and Barbara Woods (New York: Carlson, 1990), 1–11. See also Paula Giddings, *When and Where I Enter: The Impact of Black Women on Race and Sex in America* (New York: William Morrow, 1984); David J. Garrow, *The Montgomery Bus Boycott and the Women Who Started It: The Memoir of Jo Ann Gibson Robinson* (Knoxville: University of Tennessee Press, 1987); Karen Brodkin Sacks, *Caring by the Hour: Women, Work, and Organizing at Duke Medical Center* (Urbana: University of Illinois Press, 1988).

2. There are interesting parallels to the role of ministers and female members in the Baptist church. Evelyn Brooks Higginbotham, *Righteous Discontent: The Women's Movement in the Black Baptist Church, 1880–1920* (Cambridge, Mass.: Harvard University Press, 1993), ix, 49–50.

3. Judith Walzer Leavitt, "Medicine in Context: A Review Essay of the History of Medicine," *American Historical Review* 95 (December 1990): 1471–84; Edward H. Beardsley, *A History of Neglect: Health Care for Blacks and Mill Workers in the Twentieth-Century South* (Knoxville: University of Tennessee Press, 1987), 102–3, 312.

4. Darlene Clark Hine, *When the Truth Is Told: A History of Black Women's Culture and Community in Indiana, 1875–1950* (n.p.: National Council of Negro Women, 1981), 45; commentaries by James Oliver Horton and Nell Irvin Painter in *The State of Afro-American History: Past, Present, and Future*, ed. Darlene Clark Hine (Baton Rouge: Louisiana State University Press, 1986), 80–81, 133; Bart Landry, *The New Black Middle Class* (Berkeley: University of California Press, 1987), 19–21; Sharon Harley, "The Middle Class," in *Black Women in America: An Historical Encyclopedia*, vol. 2, ed. Darlene Clark Hine (New York: Carlson, 1993), 786–89.

5. Sara Lawrence Lightfoot, *Balm in Gilead: Journey of a Healer* (Reading, Mass.: Addison-Wesley, 1988), 167.

6. See Robin D. G. Kelley, " 'We Are Not What We Seem': Rethinking Black Working-Class Opposition in the Jim Crow South," *Journal of American History* 80 (June 1993): 75–112.

7. The following works have influenced my thinking on social welfare activism and the welfare state. Linda Gordon, "Family Violence, Feminism, and Social Control," *Feminist Studies* 12 (Fall 1986): 453–78; Linda Gordon, "Introduction," 24, and Nancy Fraser, "Struggle over Needs: Outline of a Socialist-Feminist Critical Theory of Late-Capitalist Political Culture," 199–225 in *Women, the State and Wel-*

fare, ed. Linda Gordon (Madison: University of Wisconsin Press, 1990); Linda Gordon, "Black and White Visions of Welfare: Women's Welfare Activism, 1890–1945," *Journal of American History* 78 (September 1991): 559–90; Patricia J. Williams, *The Alchemy of Race and Rights* (Cambridge, Mass.: Harvard University Press, 1991), 149–53.

8. Gordon, "Black and White Visions of Welfare"; Robyn Muncy, *Creating a Female Dominion in American Reform, 1890–1935* (New York: Oxford University Press, 1991); Anne Firor Scott, *Natural Allies: Women's Associations in American History* (Urbana: University of Illinois Press, 1993); Nancy A. Hewitt and Suzanne Lebsock, eds., *Visible Women: New Essays on American Activism* (Urbana: University of Illinois Press, 1993); Molly Ladd-Taylor, *Mother-Work: Women, Child Welfare, and the State, 1890–1930* (Urbana: University of Illinois Press, 1994).

9. Steven F. Lawson, "Freedom Then, Freedom Now: The Historiography of the Civil Rights Movement," *American Historical Review* 96 (April 1991): 464–65. See also Aldon D. Morris, introduction to *The Origins of the Civil Rights Movement: Black Communities Organizing for Change* (New York: Free Press, 1984); Darlene Clark Hine, "Lifting the Veil, Shattering the Silence: Black Women's History in Slavery and Freedom," in *The State of Afro-American History: Past, Present, and Future*, ed. Hine, 244.

10. On white women's health activities, see Judith Walzer Leavitt, *The Healthiest City: Milwaukee and the Politics of Health Reform* (Princeton, N.J.: Princeton University Press, 1982), chapter six; and Regina Morantz, "Making Women Modern: Middle-Class Women and Health Reform in 19th-Century America," in *Women and Health in America: Historical Readings*, ed. Judith Walzer Leavitt (Madison: University of Wisconsin Press, 1984), 346–58. On black women's health activities, see Marion M. Torchia, "The Tuberculosis Movement and the Race Question, 1890–1950," *Bulletin of the History of Medicine* 49 (Summer 1975): 152–68; Earline Rae Ferguson, "The Woman's Improvement Club of Indianapolis: Black Women Pioneers in Tuberculosis Work, 1903–1938," *Indiana Magazine of History* 84 (September 1988): 237–61; and Beardsley, *A History of Neglect*, 101–12.

11. United States Bureau of the Census, *The Social and Economic Status of the Black Population in the United States: An Historical View, 1790–1978*, Special Studies, Series P-23, No. 80 (Washington, D.C.: U.S. Government Printing Office, 1979), table 6 on "Black and White Population in Urban and Rural Areas, 1890–1980"; and Howard N. Rabinowitz, *Race Relations in the Urban South, 1865–1890* (New York: Oxford University Press, 1978), 4. See also "Farm Population Stabilizes at 5 million—2% of Nation," *Jackson Clarion-Ledger*, 14 September 1989, p. 4A.

12. John Harley Warner, "The Idea of Southern Medical Distinctiveness: Medical Knowledge and Practice in the Old South," in *Sickness and Health in America: Readings in the History of Medicine and Public Health*, ed. Judith Walzer Leavitt and Ronald L. Numbers (Madison: University of Wisconsin Press, 1985), 53–70.

13. Rabinowitz, *Race Relations in the Urban South*, xv, 31, 333.

14. Beardsley, *A History of Neglect*. See also Vanessa Northington Gamble, "The Negro Hospital Renaissance: The Black Hospital Movement, 1920–1945," in *The American General Hospital: Communities and Social Contexts*, ed. Diana Long and Janet Golden (Ithaca, N.Y.: Cornell University Press, 1989), 82–105; and David

McBride, *From TB to AIDS: Epidemics Among Urban Blacks Since 1900* (Albany: State University of New York Press, 1991).

15. Herbert Morais, *The History of the Negro in Medicine* (New York: Publishers Company for the Association for the Study of Negro Life and History, 1967). See also Todd L. Savitt, *Medicine and Slavery: The Diseases and Health Care of Blacks in Antebellum Virginia* (Urbana: University of Illinois Press, 1978); and James Jones, *Bad Blood: The Tuskegee Syphilis Experiment* (New York: Free Press, 1981).

16. Ralph Chester Williams, *The United States Public Health Service, 1798–1950* (Washington, D.C.: Commissioned Officers Association of the United States Public Health Service, 1951), 552.

17. Margaret H. Warner, "Public Health in the Old South," in *Science and Medicine in the Old South*, ed. Ronald L. Numbers and Todd L. Savitt (Baton Rouge: Louisiana State University Press, 1989), 228–29.

18. Elizabeth Barnaby Keeney, "Unless Powerful Sick: Domestic Medicine in the Old South," in *Science and Medicine in the Old South*, ed. Numbers and Savitt, 290; and Todd L. Savitt, "Black Health on the Plantation: Masters, Slaves, and Physicians," in *Science and Medicine in the Old South*, ed. Numbers and Savitt, 339.

19. Savitt, *Medicine and Slavery*, 77, 82, 246; Keeney, "Unless Powerful Sick," 276, 289, 290–91; Savitt, "Black Health on the Plantation," 347–48.

20. Savitt, *Medicine and Slavery*, 21, 27; Savitt, "Black Health on the Plantation," 327–29, 338; Nancy Krieger, "Shades of Difference: Theoretical Underpinnings of the Medical Controversy on Black/White Differences in the United States, 1830–1870," *International Journal of Health Services* 17, no. 2 (1987): 259, 262, 264, 272.

21. Jude Thomas May, "The Medical Care of Blacks in Louisiana During the Occupation and Reconstruction, 1862–1868: Its Social and Political Background" (Ph.D. diss., Tulane University, 1971), 52, 72, 154; and Rabinowitz, *Race Relations in the Urban South*, 133. See also Marshall Scott Legan, "The Evolution of Public Health Services in Mississippi, 1865–1910" (Ph.D. diss., University of Mississippi, 1968); Michael Anthony Cooke, "The Health of Blacks During Reconstruction, 1862–1870" (Ph.D. diss., University of Maryland, 1983), 1, 90; Leslie Schwalm, "The Meaning of Freedom: African-American Women and Their Transition from Slavery to Freedom in Lowcountry South Carolina" (Ph.D. diss., University of Wisconsin-Madison, 1991).

22. Cooke, "The Health of Blacks During Reconstruction," 2, 21, 27, 106; Rabinowitz, *Race Relations in the Urban South*, 122, 131, 135, 148.

23. Rabinowitz, *Race Relations in the Urban South*, 131, 133; Cooke, "The Health of Blacks During Reconstruction," 92; James O. Breeden, "Joseph Jones and Public Health in the New South," *Louisiana History* 32 (Fall 1991): 360.

24. Historians of social welfare generally point to the child welfare provisions of the early twentieth century as the first welfare program. See, for example, Ladd-Taylor, *Mother-Work*, 2.

25. May, "The Medical Care of Blacks," 52, 72, 154; Cooke, "The Health of Blacks During Reconstruction," 28, 110, 113, 158, 163; Gaines M. Foster, "The Limitations of Federal Health Care for Freedman, 1862–1868," *Journal of Southern History* 48 (August 1982): 362–64, 370.

26. Margaret Ellen Warner, "Public Health in the New South: Government,

Medicine and Society in the Control of Yellow Fever" (Ph.D. diss., Harvard University, 1983), 3, 6, 10, 16, 21, 74, 120. This material has since been published under the name Margaret Humphreys as *Yellow Fever and the South* (New Brunswick, N.J.: Rutgers University Press, 1992). See also John Duffy, "Social Impact of Disease in the Late 19th Century," in *Sickness and Health in America*, ed. Leavitt and Numbers, 414–21; John H. Ellis, *Yellow Fever and Public Health in the New South* (Lexington: University Press of Kentucky, 1992), 166.

27. Leavitt and Numbers, "Public Health Reform," *Sickness and Health*, 383; Duffy, "Social Impact of Disease in the Late 19th Century," 418; Warner, "Public Health in the New South," 23, 72; Breeden, "Joseph Jones and Public Health in the New South," 347, 352, 361; and Margaret Warner, "Local Control versus National Interest: The Debate over Southern Public Health, 1878–1884," *Journal of Southern History* 50 (August 1984): 407.

28. Warner, "Public Health in the New South," 7, 35–36, 76, 376, 190 n.22; Dennis C. Rousey, "Yellow Fever and Black Policemen in Memphis: A Post-Reconstruction Anomaly," *Journal of Southern History* 51 (August 1985): 357, 361, 365, 367; Breeden, "Joseph Jones and Public Health in the New South," 352; Ellis, *Yellow Fever and Public Health*, chapter 6.

29. Frederick L. Hoffman, *Race Traits and Tendencies of the American Negro* (New York: Published for the American Economics Association by Macmillan Co., 1896), 310–11, 329. See also McBride, *From TB to AIDS*, 16, 65; Krieger, "Shades of Difference," 275.

30. W. E. B. Du Bois, ed., *The Health Physique of the Negro American*, Atlanta University Publication no. 11 (Atlanta: Atlanta University Press, 1906), 110.

31. For example, the U.S. Supreme Court upheld segregation in its decision in *Plessy v. Ferguson* in 1896 and Mississippi led the effort for disenfranchisement when it passed its law in 1890. See August Meier, *Negro Thought in America 1880–1915: Racial Ideologies in the Age of Booker T. Washington* (Ann Arbor: University of Michigan Press, 1963); Herbert Shapiro, *White Violence and Black Response: From Reconstruction to Montgomery* (Amherst: University of Massachusetts Press, 1988); Rabinowitz, *Race Relations in the Urban South*, iii, xi, xiv.

32. See, for example, John Ettling, *The Germ of Laziness: Rockefeller Philanthropy and Public Health in the New South* (Cambridge, Mass.: Harvard University Press, 1981); and Elizabeth Etheridge, *The Butterfly Caste: A Social History of Pellagra in the South* (Westport, Conn.: Greenwood Press, 1972).

33. Etheridge, *The Butterfly Caste*, 4, 9, 13, 16, 41, 70, 120; Legan, "The Evolution of Public Health Services in Mississippi," 152; Daphne A. Roe, *A Plague of Corn: The Social History of Pellagra* (Ithaca, N.Y.: Cornell University Press, 1973), 77, 78; Bess Furman, *A Profile of the United States Public Health Service, 1798–1948* (Washington, D.C.: U.S. Government Printing Office, 1973), 300–301.

34. Ettling, *The Germ of Laziness*, 2, 3, 5, 132, 220; Etheridge, *The Butterfly Caste*, 14. While Ettling focuses on the religious methods of evangelical Christianity used by the hookworm campaign organizers, E. Richard Brown emphasizes the economic motivations of northern capitalists in promoting a healthy southern work force. E. Richard Brown, *Rockefeller Medicine Men: Medicine and Capitalism in America* (Berkeley: University of California Press, 1979).

35. Ettling, *The Germ of Laziness*; Felix Joel Underwood and Richard Noble Whitfield, *Public Health and Medical Licensure in the State of Mississippi, 1938–1947* (Jackson, Miss.: Tucker Printing House, 1951), 157–58, 262; Etheridge, *The Butterfly Caste*, 220.

36. Etheridge, *The Butterfly Caste*, 48, 59, 131.

37. Ettling, *The Germ of Laziness*, 4, 175–76.

38. Morais, *The History of the Negro in Medicine*, 86, 122; and Judith Walzer Leavitt and Ronald L. Numbers, "Sickness and Health in America: An Overview," In *Sickness and Health in America*, 5, figure 2. See also Beardsley, *A History of Neglect*, chapter 1.

39. On the history of the USPHS see Williams, *The United States Public Health Service*; Furman, *A Profile of the United States Public Health Service*; Fitzhugh Mullan, *Plagues and Politics: The Story of the United States Public Health Service* (New York: Basic Books, 1989).

40. Allan M. Brandt, *No Magic Bullet: A Social History of Venereal Disease in the United States Since 1880* (New York: Oxford University Press, 1987).

41. Richard A. Meckel, *Save the Babies: American Public Health Reform and the Prevention of Infant Mortality, 1850–1929* (Baltimore: Johns Hopkins University Press, 1990), 212; Ladd-Taylor, *Mother-Work*, chapter 6.

42. Warner, "Public Health in the New South," 379.

43. Beardsley, *A History of Neglect*, chapter 7.

44. On the parallels in the history of black education, see James D. Anderson, *The Education of Blacks in the South, 1860–1935* (Chapel Hill: University of North Carolina Press, 1988).

45. Vanessa Northington Gamble, Introduction to *Germs Have No Color Lines: Blacks and American Medicine, 1900–1949*, ed. Vanessa Northington Gamble (New York: Garland, 1989).

46. See Byllye Y. Avery, "Breathing Life into Ourselves: The Evolution of the National Black Women's Health Project," in *The Black Women's Health Book: Speaking for Ourselves*, ed. by Evelyn C. White (Seattle, Wash.: Seal Press, 1990), 4–10.

Chapter 1

1. For just a sampling of works that discuss black and/or white women's social welfare work, see W. E. B. Du Bois, ed. *Efforts for Social Betterment Among Negro Americans*, Atlanta University Publication no. 3 (Atlanta: Atlanta University Press, 1898); W. E. B. Du Bois, ed., *Efforts for Social Betterment Among Negro Americans*, Atlanta University Publication no. 14 (Atlanta: Atlanta University Press, 1909); Mary Ritter Beard, *Woman's Work in Municipalities* (New York: D. Appleton, 1915); Eleanor Flexner, *Century of Struggle*, rev. ed. (Cambridge, Mass.: Belknap Press of Harvard University Press, 1975), 184, 191; Gerda Lerner, *The Majority Finds Its Past: Placing Women in History* (New York: Oxford University Press, 1979), 67–68, 83–84; Suellen M. Hoy, "'Municipal Housekeeping': The Role of Women in Improving Urban Sanitation Practices, 1880–1917," in *Pollution and Reform in American Cities, 1870–1930*, ed. Martin V. Melosi (Austin: University of

Texas Press, 1980), 173–98; Kathleen C. Berkeley, "'Colored Ladies Also Contributed': Black Women's Activities from Benevolence to Social Welfare, 1866–1896," in *The Web of Southern Social Relations: Women, Family and Education*, ed. Walter J. Fraser, R. Frank Saunders, Jr., and Jon Wakelyn (Athens: University of Georgia Press, 1985), 181–203; Judith Walzer Leavitt, *The Healthiest City: Milwaukee and the Politics of Health Reform* (Princeton, N.J.: Princeton University Press, 1982); and Anne Firor Scott, *Natural Allies: Women's Associations in American History* (Urbana: University of Illinois Press, 1993), especially chapter 6.

2. Fannie Barrier Williams, "Club Movement Among Negro Women," in *Progress of a Race*, ed. J. W. Gibson and W. H. Crogman (Atlanta: J. L. Nichols, 1902); Elizabeth Lindsay Davis, *Lifting as They Climb* (Washington, D.C.: National Association of Colored Women, 1933); Sharon Harley and Rosalyn Terborg-Penn, eds., *The Afro-American Woman: Struggles and Images* (Port Washington, N.Y.: National University Publications, Kennikat Press, 1978); Lerner, "Community Work of Black Club Women," in *The Majority Finds Its Past*, 83–93; Darlene Clark Hine, *When the Truth Is Told: A History of Black Women's Culture and Community in Indiana, 1875–1950* (n.p.: National Council of Negro Women, 1981); Paula Giddings, *When and Where I Enter: The Impact of Black Women on Race and Sex in America* (New York: William Morrow, 1984); Susan Lynn Smith, "The Black Women's Club Movement: Self-Improvement and Sisterhood, 1890–1915" (master's thesis, University of Wisconsin-Madison, 1986); Cynthia Neverdon-Morton, *Afro-American Women of the South and the Advancement of the Race, 1895–1925* (Knoxville: University of Tennessee Press, 1989); Anne Firor Scott, "Most Invisible of All: Black Women's Voluntary Associations," *Journal of Southern History* 61 (February 1990): 3–22; Dorothy Salem, *To Better Our World: Black Women in Organized Reform, 1890–1920* (New York: Carlson, 1990), 74–78.

3. Judith Walzer Leavitt and Ronald L. Numbers, eds., *Sickness and Health in America: Readings in the History of Medicine and Public Health* (Madison: University of Wisconsin Press, 1985), 5, figure 2; Thomas McKeown, *The Modern Rise of Population* (New York: Academic Press, 1976); Thomas McKeown, *The Role of Medicine: Dream, Mirage or Nemesis?* (Princeton, N.J.: Princeton University Press, 1979); Herbert M. Morais, *The History of the Negro in Medicine* (New York: Publishers Company for the Association for the Study of Negro Life and History, 1967), chapter 5.

4. Mrs. M. M. Hubert, "Club Women's View of National Negro Health Week," *National Negro Health News* 3 (April–June 1935): 3. See also "National Association of Colored Women," *Southern Workman* 45 (September 1916): 492; Du Bois, *Efforts for Social Betterment Among Negro Americans* (1909), 47, 62, 87; Davis, *Lifting As They Climb*, 90, 125; and Emily H. Williams, "The National Association of Colored Women," *Southern Workman* 43 (September 1914): 482.

5. Elizabeth Lindsay Davis, "Votes for Philanthropy," *Crisis* 10 (August 1915): 191.

6. Fannie B. Williams, "The Negro and Public Opinion," *Voice of the Negro* 1 (January 1904): 31. See also Hine, *When the Truth Is Told*, 45.

7. Mary Church Terrell, "What Role Is the Educated Negro Woman to Play in the Uplifting of Her Race?" in *Twentieth Century Negro Literature*, ed. Daniel W. Culp (Naperville, Ill.: J. L. Nichols, 1902), 175.

8. Deborah Gray White, "The Cost of Club Work, the Price of Black Feminism," in *Visible Women: New Essays on American Activism*, ed. Nancy A. Hewitt and Suzanne Lebsock (Urbana: University of Illinois Press, 1993), 260.

9. Gerda Lerner, *Black Women in White America: A Documentary History* (New York: Random House, 1972), chapter 3; Bettina Aptheker, "Woman Suffrage and the Crusade Against Lynching, 1890–1920," in *Woman's Legacy: Essays on Race, Sex, and Class* (Amherst: University of Massachusetts Press, 1982), 53–76; Darlene Clark Hine, "Rape and the Inner Lives of Black Women in the Middle West: Preliminary Thoughts on the Culture of Dissemblance," *Signs: Journal of Women in Culture and Society* 14 (Summer 1989): 917; Hazel Carby, "'On the Threshold of Woman's Era': Lynching, Empire, and Sexuality in Black Feminist Theory," in *Race, Writing and Difference*, ed. Henry Louise Gates, Jr. (Chicago: University of Chicago Press, 1985), 301–16; White, "The Cost of Club Work," 254, 258–59.

10. Fannie Barrier Williams, "A Northern Negro's Autobiography," in *Fragments of Autobiography*, ed. Leon Stein (New York: Arno Press, 1974), 96.

11. Anna J. Cooper, "Discussion of 'The Intellectual Progress of the Colored Women of the United States since the Emancipation Proclamation,'" in *The World's Congress of Representative Women*, ed. May Wright Sewall (Chicago and New York: Rand, McNally, 1894), 711; Ellen Carol DuBois and Linda Gordon, "Seeking Ecstasy on the Battlefield: Danger and Pleasure in Nineteenth-Century Feminist Sexual Thought," *Feminist Studies* 9 (Spring 1983): 7–25; and E. Frances White, "Africa on My Mind: Gender, Counter Discourse and African-American Nationalism," *Journal of Women's History* 2 (Spring 1990): 73–97.

12. Jacqueline Jones, *Labor of Love, Labor of Sorrow: Black Women, Work, and the Family from Slavery to the Present* (New York: Basic Books, 1985), 155; and United States Bureau of the Census, *The Social and Economic Status of the Black Population in the United States: An Historical View, 1790–1978* (Washington, D.C.: U.S. Government Printing Office, 1979), 15, table 8; Edward H. Beardsley, *A History of Neglect: Health Care for Blacks and Mill Workers in the Twentieth-Century South* (Knoxville: University of Tennessee Press, 1987), 24.

13. Philip M. Hauser and Evelyn M. Kitagawa, *Local Community Fact Book for Chicago, 1950* (Chicago: Chicago Community Inventory, 1953), 2, table D; and Allan H. Spear, *Black Chicago: The Making of a Negro Ghetto, 1890–1920* (Chicago: University of Chicago Press, 1967), 12.

14. On the history of white hospitals, see Morris J. Vogel, *The Invention of the Modern Hospital, Boston, 1870–1930* (Chicago: University of Chicago Press, 1980); Charles Rosenberg, "Inward Vision and Outward Glance: The Shaping of the American Hospital, 1880–1914," *Bulletin of the History of Medicine* 53 (1979): 346–91; David Rosner, *A Once Charitable Enterprise: Hospitals and Health Care in Brooklyn and New York, 1885–1915* (Cambridge: Cambridge University Press, 1982). For an excellent overview of the history of black hospitals and extensive bibliographical information, see Vanessa Northington Gamble, *The Black Community Hospital: Contemporary Dilemmas in Historical Perspective* (New York: Garland, 1989).

15. Vanessa Northington Gamble, "The Negro Hospital Renaissance: The Black Hospital Movement, 1920–1940" (Ph.D. diss., University of Pennsylvania, 1987); Vanessa Northington Gamble, "The Negro Hospital Renaissance: The Black Hospital Movement, 1920–1945," in *The American General Hospital: Commu-*

nities and Social Contests, ed. Diana E. Long and Janet Golden (Ithaca, N.Y.: Cornell University Press, 1989), 82–105; Patricia Ellen Sloan, "A History of the Establishment and Early Development of Selected Schools of Nursing For Afro-Americans, 1886–1906" (Ph.D. diss., Teachers College, Columbia University, 1978); and Darlene Clark Hine, *Black Women in White: Racial Conflict and Cooperation in the Nursing Profession, 1890–1950* (Bloomington: Indiana University Press, 1989).

16. Hine, Introduction to *Black Women in White*; Salem, *To Better Our World*, 74–78; Stephanie J. Shaw, "Black Club Women and the Creation of the National Association of Colored Women," *Journal of Women's History* 3 (Fall 1991): 18; Scott, *Natural Allies*, 148. See also Mary Roth Walsh, "Feminist Showplace," in *Women and Health in America: Historical Readings*, ed. Judith Walzer Leavitt (Madison: University of Wisconsin Press, 1984), 392–405.

17. Theresita E. Norris, "An Historical Review of Provident Hospital," unpublished manuscript, Wisconsin State Historical Society, Madison, 1946[?]; Helen Buckler, *Daniel Hale Williams: Negro Surgeon* (New York: Pitman, 1954; reprint, 1968); Spear, *Black Chicago*; Morais, *The History of the Negro in Medicine*, 70, 74–75; Sloan, "A History of Nursing"; Hine, *Black Women in White*, 27–34; and Vanessa Northington Gamble, "The Provident Hospital Project: An Experiment in Race Relations and Medical Education," *Bulletin of the History of Medicine* 65 (Winter 1991): 457–75.

18. Dr. Williams performed the heart surgery in 1893 and the resulting publicity increased the prestige of Provident Hospital. See U. G. Dailey, "Daniel Hale Williams," *Journal of the National Medical Association* 23 (October–December 1931): 173–75; Irene Gaines, "Dr. Dan Williams: His Life," *Crisis* 39 (January 1932): 461; and Frank Lincoln Mather, ed. *Who's Who of the Colored Race: A General Biographical Dictionary of Men and Women of Colored Descent* (Chicago: F. L. Mather, 1915), 284–85.

19. Lois Wille, "Emma Reynolds — Chicago Symbol," *Chicago Daily News*, 21 January 1961 (courtesy of Provident Medical Center, Chicago).

20. Norris, "An Historical Review of Provident Hospital," 1; and Hauser and Kitagawa, *Local Community Fact Book for Chicago*, 2, table D.

21. Gamble, "The Negro Hospital Renaissance," both her dissertation and her article in *The American General Hospital*.

22. Sloan, "A History of Nursing," 85; Edward T. James, Janet Wilson James, and Paul Boyer, eds., *Notable American Women*, vol. 3 (Cambridge, Mass.: Belknap Press of Harvard University Press, 1971), 621.

23. Mrs. N. F. Mossell, *The Work of the Afro-American Woman* (1894; reprint, Freeport, N.Y.: Books for Libraries Press, 1971), 111–12; Davis, *Lifting as They Climb*, 266.

24. Buckler, *Daniel Hale Williams*, 71; Darlene Clark Hine, "From Hospital to College: Black Nurse Leaders and the Rise of Collegiate Nursing Schools," *Journal of Negro Education* 51 (Summer 1982): 222–24.

25. Adah B. Thoms, *Pathfinders: A History of the Progress of Colored Graduate Nurses* (New York: Kay Printing House, 1929), 20; Buckler, *Daniel Hale Williams*, 83; Sloan, "A History of Nursing," 114.

26. *First Annual Report of Provident Hospital and Training School* [hereinafter

PHTS] (Chicago: Desplaines Press, P. F. Pettibone, 1892), 16; Robert McMurdy, "Negro Women as Trained Nurses," *Southern Workman* 43 (January 1914): 33; George C. Hall, "Negro Hospitals," *Southern Workman* 39 (October 1910): 551; "Hospital for the Colored," *Chicago Times*, 5 May 1891, p. 2; Spear, *Black Chicago*, 31, 33; Hine, *When the Truth Is Told*, 45.

27. *PHTS, First Annual Report* (1892), 6, 29; *PHTS, Fifth Annual Report* (1896), 6–7, 14, 23; Buckler, *Daniel Hale Williams*, 70, 73; Mossell, *The Work of the Afro-American Woman*, 30, 45; Sloan, "A History of Nursing," 88; Hine, *Black Women in White*, xvii.

28. S. G. L. Dannett, *Profiles of Negro Womanhood*, vol. 2 (Yonkers, N.Y.: Negro Heritage Library, Educational Heritage, 1966), 104; Joyce Ann Elmore, "Black Nurses: Their Service and Their Struggles," *American Journal of Nursing* 76 (March 1976): 435; Sloan, "A History of Nursing," 86; Hine, *Black Women in White*, 28; and James Clark Fifield, ed., *American and Canadian Hospitals* (Minneapolis: Midwest, 1933), 291.

29. Josephine Silone Yates, "The National Association of Colored Women," *Voice of the Negro* 1 (July 1904): 286.

30. Spear, *Black Chicago*, 99.

31. "Hospital for the Colored," *Chicago Times*, p. 2; Buckler, *Daniel Hale Williams*, 70; *PHTS, Seventh Annual Report* (1898), 32; "Hospital for Colored People," *Chicago Tribune*, 5 May 1891, p. 3; Davis, *Lifting as They Climb*, 133; Emily H. Williams, "The National Association of Colored Women," *Southern Workman* 43 (August 1914): 481; and Cheryl Townsend Gilkes, " 'Together and in Harness': Women's Tradition in the Sanctified Church," *Signs: A Journal of Culture and Society* 10 (Summer 1985): 678–99.

32. *PHTS, First Annual Report* (1892), 22–28; *PHTS, Seventh Annual Report* (1898), 30–32; *PHTS, Ninth Annual Report* (1900), 34–37; and *PHTS, Twelfth Annual Report* (1903), 17–21; Buckler, *Daniel Hale Williams*, 73–75; Hine, *Black Women in White*, 35; Walsh, "Feminist Showplace," 392–405.

33. *PHTS, Fifth Annual Report* (1896), 7.

34. *PHTS, Twentieth Annual Report* (1911), 11. See also *PHTS, Fourteenth Annual Report* (1905), 11–12, 34; *PHTS, Fifteenth Annual Report* (1906), 17; *PHTS, Seventeenth Annual Report* (1908), 12; Norris, "An Historical Review of Provident Hospital," 9.

35. See Elvena Bage Tillman, "The Rights of Childhood: The National Child Welfare Movement, 1890–1919" (Ph.D. diss., University of Wisconsin-Madison, 1968); John Mayer, "Private Charities in Chicago from 1871 to 1915" (Ph.D. diss., University of Minnesota, 1978), 525; Linda Gordon, *Heroes of Their Own Lives: The Politics and History of Family Violence* (New York: Viking, 1988), chapter 3; Molly Ladd-Taylor, *Mother-Work: Women, Child Welfare, and the State, 1890–1930* (Urbana: University of Illinois, 1994), part II.

36. See Mary Church Terrell, *The Progress of Colored Women* (Washington, D.C.: Pamphlets in American History, 1898), 15; Mary Church Terrell, "What Role Is the Educated Negro Woman to Play in the Uplifting of Her Race?" in *Twentieth Century Negro Literature*, ed. David W. Culp (Naperville, Ill.: J. L. Nichols, 1902), 175.

37. By 1903 the Children's Hospital Society had established a milk station at

Provident. *PHTS, Twelfth Annual Report* (1903), 14. See also *PHTS, Nineteenth Annual Report* (1910), 12, 20, 37; *PHTS, Twentieth Annual Report* (1911), 11, 20.

38. See Kathleen D. McCarthy, *Noblesse Oblige: Charity and Cultural Philanthropy in Chicago, 1849–1929* (Chicago: University of Chicago Press, 1982), 127–28; Mayer, "Private Charities in Chicago," 283. See also Leavitt, *The Healthiest City,* chapter 5; Richard A. Meckel, *Save the Babies: American Public Health Reform and the Prevention of Infant Mortality, 1850–1929* (Baltimore: Johns Hopkins University Press, 1990), chapter 3.

39. McMurdy, "Negro Women As Trained Nurses," 34. See also *PHTS, Twentieth Annual Report* (1911), 20; Mayer, "Private Charities in Chicago," 289; Marion Hunt, "Women and Childsaving: St. Louis Children's Hospital, 1879–1979," *Bulletin of the Missouri Historical Society* 36 (January 1980): 65–79.

40. Junius B. Wood, *The Negro in Chicago* (Chicago: Chicago Daily News, 1916), 17; Hall, "Negro Hospitals," 551; St. Clair Drake, *Churches and Voluntary Associations in the Chicago Negro Community* (Chicago: Works Projects Administration, 1940); Spear, *Black Chicago,* 97; August Meier, *Negro Thought in America, 1880–1915: Racial Ideologies in the Age of Booker T. Washington* (Ann Arbor: University of Michigan Press, 1963), 134.

41. Neverdon-Morton, *Afro-American Women of the South,* chapter 6; Salem, *To Better Our World,* 89–90; Lerner, *Majority Finds Its Past,* 84–85.

42. Monroe Work, "How Tuskegee Has Improved a Black Belt County," [1909?], p. 8, box 3, Monroe Nathan Work Papers, Hollis Burke Frissell Library, Tuskegee University, Tuskegee, Ala.; "Tuskegee Woman's Club," *National Notes* 30 (January 1928): 8. On teachers see Sharon Harley, "Beyond the Classroom: The Organizational Lives of Black Female Educators in the District of Columbia, 1890–1930," *Journal of Negro Education* 51 (Summer 1982): 256; Jones, *Labor of Love, Labor of Sorrow,* 143–44; Tullia Kay Brown Hamilton, "The National Association of Colored Women, 1896–1920" (Ph.D. diss., Emory University, 1978), 27, 45, 130; Neverdon-Morton, *Afro-American Women of the South,* 133, 136.

43. Finding aids folder, Margaret Murray Washington Papers, Hollis Burke Frissell Library, Tuskegee University, Tuskegee, Ala.; *Crisis* (August 1925): 191, in box 132A; Installation Ceremonies, 4 October 1972, Alabama Women's Hall of Fame, box 132, Margaret Murray Washington Papers.

44. Lerner, *Majority Finds Its Past,* 84; Lerner, *Black Women in White America,* 75–82, 132–34; Evelyn Brooks Barnett, "Nannie Burroughs and the Education of Black Women," in *The Afro-American Woman: Struggles and Images,* ed. Sharon Harley and Rosalyn Terborg-Penn (Port Washington, N.Y.: National University Publications, Kennikat Press, 1978), 98–101; Patricia Bell-Scott, "Black Women's Higher Education: Our Legacy," *Sage* 1 (Spring 1984): 8–11; Neverdon-Morton, *Afro-American Women of the South.*

45. Florence L. Lattimore, "The Palace of Delight at Hampton," *Survey* 33 (March 6, 1915): 625.

46. Work, "How Tuskegee Has Improved a Black Belt County," 18.

47. Thomas Monroe Campbell, *The Movable School Goes to the Negro Farmer* (Tuskegee, Ala.: Tuskegee Institute Press, 1936; reprint, New York: Arno Press and the New York Times, 1969), 84–85, 101–2; Louis Harlan, *Booker T. Washington: The Wizard of Tuskegee, 1901–1915* (New York: Oxford University Press, 1983), 206.

48. Campbell, *The Movable School*, 82–85; T. M. Campbell, "The Movable School in Agricultural Extension Work," in *Proceedings of Session on Negro Social Work*, 9 April 1929, 15 (located in box 1, Work Papers); Neverdon-Morton, *Afro-American Women of the South*, 123–26; and Paul Jefferson, "Working Notes on the Prehistory of Black Sociology: The Tuskegee Negro Conference," *Knowledge and Society: Studies in the Sociology of Culture Past and Present* 6 (1986): 134–36 (courtesy of Alfred Skerpan). *Southern Letter*, published by Tuskegee Institute, contains many references to these annual conferences.

49. Campbell, *The Movable School*, 85–86.

50. Work, "How Tuskegee Has Improved a Black Belt County," 9. See also "Synopsis of the Lecture by Mrs. Booker T. Washington, on The Organizing of Women's Clubs" (author unknown), box 132A, Margaret Washington Papers.

51. Mrs. Booker T. Washington, "The Negro Home," address presented at the Interracial Conference in Memphis, October 1920, published by the Woman's Missionary Council, finding aids folder, Margaret Washington Papers.

52. Washington, "The Negro Home." See also Neverdon-Morton, *Afro-American Women of the South*, 133.

53. Terrell, "What Role Is the Educated Negro Woman to Play," 172.

54. Sarah Dudley Pettey, "What Role Is the Educated Negro Woman to Play in the Uplifting of Her Race?" in *Twentieth Century Negro Literature*, ed. David W. Culp (Naperville, Ill.: J. L. Nichols, 1902), 183.

55. John A. Kenney, *The Negro in Medicine* (John A. Kenney, 1912), 59. See also "Synopsis of the Lecture by Mrs. Booker T. Washington"; "National Association of Colored Women," *Southern Workman* 45 (September 1916): 492; Thoms, *Pathfinders*, 184.

56. "Synopsis of the Lecture by Mrs. Booker T. Washington."

57. Hope was active in the National Association of Colored Women, the National Council of Negro Women, the International Council of Women of the Darker Races, the Commission on Interracial Cooperation, the National Urban League, the YWCA, and the NAACP. See Jacqueline Anne Rouse, *Lugenia Burns Hope: Black Southern Reformer* (Athens: University of Georgia Press, 1989).

58. Rouse, *Lugenia Burns Hope*, 70. See also chapter 4. Information on the Neighborhood Union, one of the more thoroughly studied black women's community organizations, can be found also in Lerner, *Black Women in White America*, 497–512; Lerner, *The Majority Finds Its Past*, 88–92; Beardsley, *A History of Neglect*, 104–8; and Neverdon-Morton, *Afro-American Women of the South*, 145–62.

59. Stuart Galishoff, "Germs Know No Color Line: Black Health and Public Policy in Atlanta, 1900–1918," *Journal of the History of Medicine and Allied Science* 40 (January 1985): 27, 29; Howard N. Rabinowitz, *Race Relations in the Urban South, 1865–1890* (New York: Oxford University Press, 1978), 97, 120–22; Jones, *Labor of Love, Labor of Sorrow*, 123.

60. George Rosen, "The First Neighborhood Health Center Movement: Its Rise and Fall," in *Sickness and Health in America*, ed. Leavitt and Numbers, 475–89; and Leavitt, *The Healthiest City*. See also Marian Strong, "A Health Center on Wheels," *Wisconsin Magazine* 1 (March 1923): 25–27.

61. "Atlanta's Public Health Program," typescript, box A6, general office file, National Urban League Southern Regional Division Collection, Library of Con-

gress, Washington, D.C.; Lerner, *Black Women in White America*, 501–9; Rouse, *Lugenia Burns Hope*, chapter 4.

62. Beardsley, *A History of Neglect*, 105; Neverdon-Morton, *Afro-American Women of the South*, 160; *Proceedings of the National Negro Business League* (1917), 66, located at Hollis Burke Frissell Library, Tuskegee University.

63. Mary Fitzbutler Waring, M.D., "Sanitation," *National Association Notes* (April–May 1917): 8–9. See also *National Notes*, vol. 16 (November 1913): 12, and vol. 26 (November 1923): 8; W. Montague Cobb, "Henry Fitzbutler," *Journal of the National Medical Association* 44 (September 1952): 403–7; "Dr. M. Fitzbutler Waring," *Who's Who in Colored America*, 6th ed., ed. Thomas Yenser (New York: Thomas Yenser, 1944), 540.

64. Secretary for the Mayor of Atlanta to Jesse Thomas, 5 April 1922, and other correspondence for the 1922 Atlanta Clean-Up Campaign, box A6, general office file, National Urban League Southern Regional Division; Mary Dickinson, Executive Secretary of the Tuberculosis Association of Atlanta, to Robert Moton, 19 March 1926, file cabinet 3, drawer 2, Department of Records and Research Collection, Hollis Burke Frissell Library, Tuskegee University, Tuskegee, Ala.

65. Proceedings of the Negro Health Week Planning Meeting at Tuskegee University, 20 January 1927, box 18, Thomas Monroe Campbell Papers, Hollis Burke Frissell Library, Tuskegee University, Tuskegee, Ala.; Atlanta Health Week Report, 1927, box 132, Robert Russa Moton Papers, Hollis Burke Frissell Library, Tuskegee University, Tuskegee, Ala.; *Proceedings of the National Negro Business League* (1917), 64; Rouse, *Lugenia Burns Hope*, 81; and Neverdon-Morton, *Afro-American Women of the South*, 160–63.

66. Forrester B. Washington to Albon Holsey, 3 May 1929. See also Atlanta Health Week Report, 1929, file cabinet 3, drawer 1, Department of Records and Research Collection.

67. Forrester B. Washington to Albon Holsey, 3 May 1929, Department of Records and Research Collection.

68. Forrester B. Washington to Albon Holsey, 3 May 1929, and Atlanta Health Week Report, 1929, Department of Records and Research Collection; Lerner, *Black Women in White America*, 506; and George Rosen, *A History of Public Health* (New York: MD Publications, 1958), 382.

69. David McBride, *From TB to AIDS: Epidemics among Urban Blacks since 1900* (Albany: State University of New York Press, 1991), 69; Beardsley, *A History of Neglect*, 24, 101–2.

Chapter 2

1. C. E. A. Winslow, *The Evolution and Significance of the Modern Public Health Campaign* (New Haven, Conn.: Yale University Press, 1923); Judith Walzer Leavitt, *The Healthiest City: Milwaukee and the Politics of Health Reform* (Princeton, N.J.: Princeton University Press, 1982), 204, 228; Barbara Gutmann Rosenkrantz, *Public Health and the State: Changing Views in Massachusetts, 1842–1936* (Cambridge, Mass.: Harvard University Press, 1972), 130.

2. Charlotte Hawkins Brown, "Cooperation Between White and Colored Women," *Missionary Review of the World* 45 (June 1922): 484–87; Louis Harlan, *Booker T. Washington: The Wizard of Tuskegee, 1901–1915* (New York: Oxford University Press, 1983); Cynthia Neverdon-Morton, *Afro-American Women of the South and the Advancement of the Race, 1895–1925* (Knoxville: University of Tennessee Press, 1989), 185, 226–33.

3. Monroe Nathan Work, as told to Lewis W. Jones, 15 May 1932, typescript "Monroe Nathan Work," finding aids folder, Monroe Work Papers, Hollis Burke Frissell Library, Tuskegee University, Tuskegee, Ala.

4. Patricia J. Williams, *The Alchemy of Race and Rights* (Cambridge, Mass.: Harvard University Press, 1991), chapter 8, especially 149, 151–52; Nancy Fraser, "Struggle Over Needs: Outline of a Socialist-Feminist Critical Theory of Late-Capitalist Political Culture," in *Women, the State, and Welfare*, ed. Linda Gordon (Madison: University of Wisconsin Press, 1990), 199, 202, 221.

5. Frederick L. Hoffman, *Race Traits and Tendencies of the American Negro* (New York: Published for the American Economics Association by Macmillan Co., 1896), 311, 329.

6. James D. Anderson, *The Education of Blacks in the South, 1860–1935* (Chapel Hill: University of North Carolina Press, 1988), chapter 5; Vanessa Northington Gamble, "The Negro Hospital Renaissance: The Black Hospital Movement, 1920–1940" (Ph.D. diss., University of Pennsylvania, 1987); Jessie M. Rodrique, "The Black Community and the Birth-Control Movement," in *Unequal Sisters: A Multicultural Reader in U.S. Women's History*, ed. Ellen Carol DuBois and Vicki L. Ruiz (New York: Routledge, 1990), 333–44.

7. Eugene Kinckle Jones, "The Negro's Struggle for Health," *National Conference of Social Work Proceedings* (1923), 72.

8. Anderson, *The Education of Blacks*, 106.

9. See August Meier, *Negro Thought in America, 1880–1915: Racial Ideologies in the Age of Booker T. Washington* (Ann Arbor: University of Michigan Press, 1963). Textbooks have repeated this characterization. See Bernard Bailyn et al., eds., *The Great Republic: A History of the American People*, vol. 2 (Lexington, Mass.: D. C. Heath and Co., 1981), 686–88.

10. W. Montague Cobb, "Fifty Years of Progress in Health," *Pittsburgh Courier* (1950), 4, located at Health Sciences Library, Howard University, Washington, D.C. See also Anderson, *The Education of Blacks*, 102–3.

11. W. E. B. Du Bois, *The Autobiography of W. E. B. Du Bois* (New York: International Publishers, 1968), 236–37; Cincinnati Health Week Report, 1927, box 132, general correspondence, Robert Russa Moton Papers, Hollis Burke Frissell Library, Tuskegee University, Tuskegee, Ala.; Harlan, *Booker T. Washington: Wizard*, ix, 417; Anderson, *The Education of Blacks*, 104; Meier, *Negro Thought in America*, 196. See also Mrs. Jessie Guzman, an employee of Tuskegee Institute since the 1920s and Monroe Work's successor as director of the Department of Records and Research at Tuskegee Institute, interviewed by the author, tape recording, Tuskegee, Ala., 10 September 1989.

12. Virginia Health Bulletin, "Handbook of Health for Colored People," vol. 6, 10 April 1914, Negro Organization Society (microfilm reel 61, special correspon-

dence, Booker T. Washington Papers, Manuscript Division, Library of Congress, Washington, D.C.); "The Negro Organization Society," *Southern Workman* 43 (December 1914): 651–53; "Better Health for Negroes," *Southern Workman* 44 (January 1915): 9–11; "Negro Organization Society," *Southern Workman* 44 (April 1915): 202–3; *Journal of the National Medical Association* 6 (January–March 1914): 68–69; *Journal of the National Medical Association* 7 (January–March 1915): 51–54; *Survey* 34 (15 May 1915): 158; Robert R. Moton, *Finding a Way Out: An Autobiography* (Garden City, N.Y.: Doubleday, Page, 1921), 169, 172, 177; Meier, *Negro Thought in America*, 123; Neverdon-Morton, *Afro-American Women of the South*, 119–20.

13. Moton, *Finding a Way Out*, 76.

14. Linda O. McMurry, *Recorder of the Black Experience: A Biography of Monroe Nathan Work* (Baton Rouge: Louisiana State University Press, 1985), 7, 28, 34–38, 40–41, 52, 112. For information on the Georgia health campaign, see Monroe N. Work, "A Health Week in Savannah Georgia in 1905," box 2, Work Papers.

15. George Rosen, *A History of Public Health* (New York: MD Publications, 1958), 259, 395.

16. McMurry, *Recorder of the Black Experience*, 52, see also 21, 28, 96.

17. Robert Moton's secretary to Allen Clark, 10 October 1922, box 89, general correspondence, Moton Papers; newsclipping from the *Montgomery Advertiser*, 18 January 1924, box 1, and Program for 1924 Tuskegee Negro Conference, box 6, Tuskegee Institute Extension Service Collection, Hollis Burke Frissell Library, Tuskegee University, Tuskegee, Ala.; and McMurry, *Recorder of the Black Experience*, 113.

18. Albon Holsey's statement, Proceedings of the Negro Health Week Planning Meeting, Washington, D.C., 1 November 1926, file cabinet 3, drawer 1, Department of Records and Research Collection, Hollis Burke Frissell Library, Tuskegee University, Tuskegee, Ala., p. 14.

19. Monroe Work, "Life Span of Negroes in Past Ten Years Increased by Five Years: National Negro Health Week One of the Most Important Factors in this Improvement," box 4, p. 1, Work Papers. See also Monroe N. Work, "The South and the Conservation of Negro Health," galley proof section of 1914–15 edition of the *Negro Year Book*, box 11, Work Papers; Monroe Work, "The Economic Waste of Sickness," paper presented at health conference in Gulfside, Miss., 5 June 1929, box 4, Work Papers; Hoffman, *Race Traits and Tendencies*, 329.

20. Booker T. Washington to Robert Moton, 25 November 1914, microfilm reel 61, special correspondence, Washington Papers.

21. Robert Moton to Booker T. Washington, 15 December 1914, microfilm reel 61, special correspondence, Washington Papers; Anson Phelps Stokes to Booker T. Washington, 24 November 1914, microfilm reel 79, special correspondence, Washington Papers; Harlan, *Booker T. Washington: Wizard*, 235.

22. Galley proof, "A Great National Health Week to Be Observed from March 21st to 27th, 1915," box 943, Washington Papers.

23. The sixteen states were Georgia, South Carolina, North Carolina, Tennessee, Kentucky, Alabama, Mississippi, Oklahoma, Missouri, Texas, Louisiana, Virginia, Maryland, Pennsylvania, New York, and Illinois. See the hundreds of news stories on Negro Health Week in the Tuskegee Institute News Clippings File,

Health Week 1915; galley proof, "A Great National Health Week," and newsclippings and other materials located in box 943, Washington Papers; Booker T. Washington, "First Call for National Negro Health Week," form letter, 1 February 1915, file cabinet 6, drawer 1, Department of Records and Research Collection. Correspondence reporting on health week activities includes Mr. F. Nichols, Ocean Springs, Miss., to Tuskegee Institute, 29 March 1915; and Eugene Kinckle Jones, New York City, to Booker T. Washington, 20 May 1915, box 510, general correspondence, Washington Papers.

24. "Negroes Flock to Health Exhibition," *Baltimore News*, 25 March 1915, Tuskegee Institute News Clippings File; Harlan, *Booker T. Washington: Wizard*, 235.

25. Harlan, *Booker T. Washington: Wizard*, 427, 425.

26. For discussion in the black press, including the St. Louis newspaper, see the Tuskegee Institute News Clippings File, Health Week 1915.

27. Vanessa Northington Gamble, ed., *Germs Have No Color Line: Blacks and American Medicine, 1900–1940* (New York: Garland, 1989).

28. Robert Moton, Proceedings of the Negro Health Week Planning Meeting, 1 November 1926.

29. Algernon B. Jackson, "The Need of Health Education Among Negroes," *Opportunity* 2 (August 1924): 235–40 (courtesy of Leslie Schwalm).

30. Robert Moton, "Nationalizing the Negro Organization Society Movement," in *Proceedings of the National Negro Business League*, 19th annual convention (Boston, 1915), 159–60.

31. Quoted in Stuart Galishoff, "Germs Know No Color Line: Black Health and Public Policy in Atlanta, 1900–1918," *Journal of the History of Medicine and Allied Sciences* 40 (January 1985): 29. I have repeated the lower-case spelling of "Negro" as in the original.

32. Quoted in Galishoff, "Germs Know No Color Line," 29.

33. Booker T. Washington, "What Co-operation Can Accomplish," *Southern Workman* 43 (December 1914): 661. He delivered this speech before the Negro Organization Society in Norfolk, Va., 12 November 1914.

34. Harlan, *Booker T. Washington: Wizard*, 236.

35. Nannie Helen Burroughs to Emmett Scott, 17 July 1917, and Scott to Burroughs, 21 July 1917, box 14, general correspondence, Moton Papers. See also galley proof, "Conservation of Negro Health," call for 1917 Negro Health Week, box 943, Washington Papers; *Southern Letter* 34 (March 1917): 1.

36. Moton, *Finding a Way Out*, chapter 11; and *Southern Letter* (January 1919): 3. On the influenza epidemic see Leavitt, *The Healthiest City*, chapter 7; K. David Patterson and Gerald F. Pyle, "The Geography and Mortality of the 1918 Influenza Pandemic," *Bulletin of the History of Medicine* 65 (Spring 1991): 4–21.

37. The black organizations that supported Negro Health Week were the National Negro Business League, Circle for Negro Relief (New York), National Association of Colored Women, National Association of Colored Graduate Nurses, National Medical Association, National Urban League, North Carolina Mutual Life Insurance Company, and National Association of Teachers in Colored Schools. See correspondence from Moton to these organizations throughout the 1920s, such as the file on "affiliating agencies" in drawer 2, file cabinet 3, Department of Records

and Research Collection. See also the list of sponsors printed on the health week bulletins in 1922 and 1923: "Program of the Eighth Annual National Negro Health Week, April 2 to 8, 1922" (Washington, D.C.: U.S. Government Printing Office, 1922); "National Negro Health Week, April 1 to 7, 1923," box 89, general correspondence, Moton Papers. See also specific histories of these organizations, such as Thelma D. Perry, *History of the American Teachers Association* (Washington, D.C.: National Education Association, 1975), chapter 8 (courtesy of Michael Fultz).

38. *New York Urban League, Report 1920*, vol. 3 (January 1921) and Eugene K. Jones, Report of the Executive Secretary of the National Urban League to the Executive Board, 23 May 1921, box 79, general correspondence, Moton Papers; Jones to Robert Moton, 26 January 1923, and Jones form letter to "friends," 5 June 1923, box 90, general correspondence, Moton Papers.

39. The white organizations that supported black health week during the 1920s included the American Social Hygiene Association, National Child Welfare Association, Child Health Organization, Texas Public Health Association, Clean-up and Paint-up Campaign Bureau, Commission on Interracial Cooperation, National Tuberculosis Association, National Health Council, National Organization for Public Health Nursing, International Health Board of the Rockefeller Foundation, American Red Cross, National Health Council, YMCA, YWCA, and Cleanliness Institute. For an example of the interactions between white organizations and Tuskegee Institute, see Philip Klein, Associate Director of field studies for the American Red Cross, to Monroe Work, 8 February 1921, and W. Frank Persons to Monroe Work, 23 February 1921, box 18, Thomas M. Campbell Papers, Hollis Burke Frissell Library, Tuskegee University, Tuskegee, Ala. *The Red Cross Courier* advertised Negro Health Week to members of the American Red Cross during the 1920s (courtesy of Mary D. Doering, Curator, National Headquarters of the American Red Cross, Washington, D.C.).

40. Proceedings of the Negro Health Week Planning Meeting, Tuskegee Institute, January 1927.

41. Proceedings of the National Negro Health Week Planning Meeting, 11 November 1926; Robert Moton to Hugh Cumming, 23 September 1927, box 138, general correspondence, Moton Papers; "Thirteenth Annual Negro Health Week To Be Observed April 3–10," call for health week, box 132, general correspondence, Moton Papers; and form letter from Moton to participating agencies with planning meeting agenda items, 8 October 1928, file cabinet 3, drawer 1, Department of Records and Research Collection.

42. In April 1916, Emmett Scott first proposed the idea of honoring Washington, which the executive committee of the National Negro Business League agreed to in 1919. McMurry claims that the idea actually belonged to Monroe Work. Emmett Scott to Dr. A. M. Brown, 12 April 1916, box 1, and Robert Moton to F. Rivers Barnwell, 20 January 1920, box 59, general correspondence, Moton Papers; *Southern Letter* 37 (May 1920): 3; and McMurry, *Recorder of the Black Experience*, 115.

43. Monroe Work, "An Autobiographical Sketch," box 1, Work Papers, 5.

44. Robert Moton to Roscoe Brown, 2 October 1920, box 59, general corre-

spondence, Moton Papers; Robert Moton to Hugh Cumming, 24 January 1921, box 66, general correspondence, Moton Papers; Gertrude H. Bowling, *Public Health Nurse* 19 (February 1927): 85. See also Rosen, *A History of Public Health*, 382.

45. Proceedings of the Negro Health Week Planning Meeting, 1 November 1926, pp. 8–9; Robert Moton to T. E. Edwards, National Health Council, 11 February 1926, box 132, general correspondence, Moton Papers; *Southern Letter* 43 (March 1927): 1; Robert Moton to Roscoe Brown, 22 September 1928, file cabinet 3, drawer 1, Department of Records and Research Collection; Robert Moton to Superintendent of Documents, U.S. Government Printing Office, 12 December 1928, box 156, general correspondence, Moton Papers; McMurry, *Recorder of the Black Experience*, 115–16.

46. Robert Moton to Surgeon General Cumming, 6 January 1926, file cabinet 3, drawer 2, Department of Records and Research Collection. The first mention of National Negro Health Week by the Annual Report of the Surgeon General was in 1924. *Annual Report of the Surgeon General of the Public Health Service of the United States for the Fiscal Year 1924* [hereinafter *Annual Report of the USPHS*] (Washington, D.C.: U.S. Government Printing Office, 1924), 2

47. I have extrapolated these goals through analysis of the proceedings of national health week planning meetings. See, for example, Proceedings of the Negro Health Week Planning Meeting, Washington, D.C., 1 November 1926, file cabinet 3, drawer 1, Department of Records and Research Collection.

48. Robert Moton to Hugh Cumming, 22 January 1923, box 80, general correspondence, Moton Papers.

49. Jesse O. Thomas to Robert Moton, 26 January 1923, box 90, general correspondence, Moton Papers.

50. Jesse O. Thomas to Robert Moton, 26 January 1923, box 90, general correspondence, Moton Papers. See also Proceedings of Negro Health Week Planning Meeting, 1 November 1926.

51. Ronald L. Numbers, "The Third Party: Health Insurance in America," in *Sickness and Health in America: Readings in the History of Medicine and Public Health*, ed. Judith Walzer Leavitt and Ronald L. Numbers (Madison: University of Wisconsin Press, 1985), 238; and Ronald Numbers, *Almost Persuaded: American Physicians and Compulsory Health Insurance, 1912–1920* (Baltimore: Johns Hopkins University Press, 1978).

52. Moton, Proceedings of Negro Health Week planning meeting, 1 November 1926.

53. Work, "An Autobiographical Sketch," 5.

54. Bernice Scott to Albon Holsey, 6 March 1929, file cabinet 3, drawer 1, Department of Records and Research Collection. See also Barbara Melosh, *"The Physician's Hand": Work Culture and Conflict in American Nursing* (Philadelphia: Temple University Press, 1982), title of chapter 4.

55. Richard L. Bushman and Claudia L. Bushman, "The Early History of Cleanliness in America," *Journal of American History* 74 (March 1988): 1213–38.

56. Gert H. Brieger, "Sanitary Reform in New York City: Stephen Smith and the Passage of the Metropolitan Health Bill," 399–413, and Judith Walzer Leavitt

and Ronald L. Numbers, "Changing Public Health Concerns," 473, in *Sickness and Health in America*, ed. Leavitt and Numbers; Paul Starr, *The Social Transformation of American Medicine* (New York: Basic Books, 1982), part I, chapter 5.

57. "Negroes Co-operate in Movement to Make Knoxville Cleaner." See also additional descriptions of early Negro Health Week programs in Tuskegee Institute News Clippings File, Health Week 1915; and descriptions in box 943, Washington Papers.

58. Mrs. M. M. Hubert, "Club Women's View of National Negro Health Week," *National Negro Health News* 3 (April–June 1935): 5.

59. Dr. H. S. Mustard, Assistant Commissioner of the Department of Public Health, Tennessee, to Robert Moton, 10 February 1930, and Nashville Health Week Report, 1930, submitted by James H. Robinson, Executive Secretary of Health Week Committee, file cabinet 3, drawer 2, Department of Records and Research Collection.

60. Burroughs quoted in Anne Firor Scott, "Most Invisible of All: Black Women's Voluntary Associations," *Journal of Southern History* 56 (February 1990): 13. See also Evelyn Brooks Barnett, "Nannie Burroughs and the Education of Black Women," in *The Afro-American Woman: Struggles and Images*, ed. Sharon Harley and Rosalyn Terborg-Penn (Port Washington, N.Y.: University Publications, Kennikat Press, 1978), 97–108. On Margaret Murray Washington, see Jacqueline Anne Rouse, *Lugenia Burns Hope: Black Southern Reformer* (Athens: University of Georgia Press, 1989), 8; Neverdon-Morton, *Afro-American Women of the South*, 132–37.

61. "The Niagara Movement: Declaration of Principles, 1905," box 2, Work Papers. See also Elliott Rudwick, "The Niagara Movement," in *The Making of Black America*, vol. 2, ed. August Meier and Elliott Rudwick (New York: Atheneum, 1969), 131–48.

62. Galley proof, "Judges Selected to Award Prizes to Healthy Cities," box 132, general correspondence, Moton Papers. Fauset is mentioned as a judge in *Southern Letter* 44 (September 1928): 4. For information on Dunbar-Nelson, see Gloria T. Hull, ed., *Give Us Each Day: The Diary of Alice Dunbar-Nelson* (New York: W. W. Norton, 1984).

63. See material in box 195, general files, 1924–35, Record Group 90, United States Public Health Service (USPHS), National Archives, Washington, D.C.; "Reports of the National 'Clean Up and Paint Up Campaign,' 1922," box 89, general correspondence, Moton Papers.

64. Memo to Monroe Work, 29 June 1929, file cabinet 2, drawer 1, Department of Records and Research Collection; *Southern Letter* 44 (September 1928): 4.

65. Work, "The Economic Waste of Sickness," 7.

66. Ruth Evelyn Henderson to Robert Moton, 2 May 1928, file cabinet 3, drawer 1, Department of Records and Research Collection.

67. F. Rivers Barnwell to Monroe Work, 26 December 1928, and Barnwell to Work, 10 May 1929, file cabinet 3, drawer 1, Department of Records and Research Collection.

68. Robert Moton to Grace Abbott, 4 March 1922, box 198, Central File, 1921–1924, Record Group 102, Children's Bureau, National Archives, Washington, D.C. See also Robert Moton to Grace Abbott, 15 December 1921, and Memoran-

dum from Anna Rude, M.D., director of the Division of Hygiene, to Grace Abbott, 5 January 1921, box 225, Central File, 1921–1924, Record Group 102, Children's Bureau; *National Association Notes* (April 1918): 3; Molly Ladd-Taylor, *Raising a Baby the Government Way: Mothers' Letters to the Children's Bureau* (New Brunswick, N.J.: Rutgers University Press, 1986).

69. S. W. Welch form letter to southern state health officers, 5 March 1925, file cabinet 3, drawer 2, Department of Records and Research Collection.

70. W. F. Draper to Monroe Work, 5 March 1926, box 74, General Files, 1924–1935, Record Group 90, USPHS. See also Proceedings of the Negro Health Week Planning Meeting, 1 November 1926, box 59, general correspondence, Moton Papers; Alabama Health Officer to Robert Moton, 6 February 1929, file cabinet 3, drawer 1, Department of Records and Research Collection.

71. George Brown Tindall, *The Emergence of the New South, 1913–1945* (Baton Rouge: Louisiana State University Press and the Littlefield Fund for Southern History of the University of Texas, 1967), 69.

72. C. W. Garrison to Robert Moton, 6 February 1929, file cabinet 3, drawer 1, Department of Records and Research Collection.

73. J. T. Irby to Tuskegee Institute, 16 March 1929, file cabinet 3, drawer 1, Department of Records and Research Collection.

74. F. Papenhausen to Robert Moton, 18 March 1929, file cabinet 3, drawer 1, Department of Records and Research Collection.

75. Mrs. W. L. Thompson to Tuskegee Institute, 16 March 1929, and Robert Moton to Thompson, 20 March 1929, file cabinet 3, drawer 1, Department of Records and Research. See also *National Notes* 17 (May–June 1915): 23.

76. Robert Moton to Hugh Cumming, 22 January 1923, box 80, general correspondence, Moton Papers.

77. James Bond to Robert Moton, 4 May 1927, and Louisville Health Week Report, 1927, box 132, general correspondence, Moton Papers.

78. Cincinnati Health Week Report, 1927, submitted by James H. Robinson, box 132, general correspondence, Moton Papers. See also John M. Ragland to Monroe Work, 15 July 1929, file cabinet 3, drawer 1, Department of Records and Research Collection.

79. The Department of Records and Research Collection at Tuskegee University is a rich reservoir of material about black health activism. For just a sampling of the available correspondence, see Mary Foster McDavid, Department of Education, Alabama, to Monroe Work, 10 February 1930, file cabinet 3, drawer 2; Helen Hewlett, Home Demonstration Agent in charge of Negro work, Gulfport, Miss., to Robert Moton, 15 March 1930, file cabinet 3, drawer 1; Mary L. Ray, Home Demonstration Agent, Little Rock, Ark., to Tuskegee Institute, 24 February 1930, file cabinet 3, drawer 2.

80. There is much evidence of the participation of local chapters of these national organizations. For a brief sampling, see Mary M. Vickens, Ashbury Park, N.J., branch of the NAACP, to Tuskegee Institute, 1933, file cabinet 3, drawer 4, Department of Records and Research Collection; reports from sixteen cities on health week in Eugene Kinckle Jones, "Statements on the Health Programs of Some of the Affiliated Branches of the National Urban League," 18 September 1940, box

10, National Urban League Records, Series 5, Public Relations Dept., C. Historical Information File, Library of Congress, Washington, D.C.; *Red Cross Courier* for March 1944, April 1945, April 1946, April 1947.

81. See, for example, Monroe Work to Mrs. M. M. Hubert, Chair of Civic Committee of City Federation of Colored Women's Clubs, Jackson, Miss., 29 January 1932, file cabinet 3, drawer 3; and Mrs. Nellie Bird, Frances Harper Woman's Club, Ithaca, N.Y., to Tuskegee Institute, 18 March 1930, file cabinet 3, drawer 1, Department of Records and Research Collection.

82. Letter to Robert Moton, 22 February 1930, and Lodie M. Biggs to Moton, 11 January 1930, file cabinet 3, drawer 2, Department of Records and Research Collection.

83. Seattle, Wash., Health Week Report, 1929, submitted by Mrs. Gordon Carter, file cabinet 3, drawer 2, Department of Records and Research Collection.

84. William George Tyson, "The Incidence of Syphilis in Negroes," *Journal of the National Medical Association* 27 (February 1935): 8–9.

85. Hassie A. Towler, "Health Education in Ward 9," *Public Health Nurse* 21 (August 1929): 417–18.

86. Detroit Health Week Report, 28 April 1930, file cabinet 3, drawer 2, Department of Records and Research Collection.

87. Waco, Tex., Health Week Report, 1929, submitted by Mrs. R. V. Estelle, President of the Volunteer Health League, file cabinet 2, drawer 1, Department of Records and Research Collection.

88. Thomasville, Ala., Health Week Report, 1929, submitted by Mrs. M. N. Dickinson; Dickinson to Robert Moton, 12 April 1929; Monroe Work to Dickinson, 18 April 1929, file cabinet 3, drawer 1, Department of Records and Research Collection.

89. Chicago Health Week Report, 1929, part I, 8–9, file cabinet 3, drawer 1, Department of Records and Research Collection.

90. H. R. Crawford, YMCA, to Monroe Work, 20 July 1929, file cabinet 3, drawer 1, Department of Records and Research Collection.

91. Chicago Health Week Report, part I, 3.

92. Chicago Health Week Report, part I, 4–6, and part II, 7.

93. Chicago Health Week Report.

94. Chicago Health Week Report, part II, 12, 15, 25–26.

95. Chicago Health Week Report, part II, 10, 16–21.

96. Chicago Health Week Report, part II, 16–21.

97. Work, "The Economic Waste of Sickness."

98. The largest number of campaigns were held in Alabama, Georgia, Kentucky, Texas, and Virginia. Chart, "Negro Health Week Observance for the six years 1925–30," file cabinet 3, drawer 2, Department of Records and Research Collection. For information on Negro Health Week in West Africa see *Southern Letter* 43 (March 1927): 4; on Canada see *Southern Letter* 45 (March–April 1929): 3.

99. Monroe Work, in *Proceedings of the National Negro Business League* (1924), 89.

100. Hugh Cumming to Robert Moton, 25 October 1929, and Proceedings of the Negro Health Week Planning Meeting, Washington, D.C., 19 October 1929, file

cabinet 3, drawer 1, Department of Records and Research Collection. See also Roscoe Brown to Robert Moton, 31 December 1929, box 156, general correspondence, Moton Papers.

101. *Southern Letter* 43 (August 1927): 2–3; Harlan, *Booker T. Washington: Wizard*, 197.

102. Robert Moton to Hugh Cumming, 14 November 1929, file cabinet 3, drawer 1, Department of Records and Research Collection.

Chapter 3

1. Edward H. Beardsley, *A History of Neglect: Health Care for Blacks and Mill Workers in the Twentieth-Century South* (Knoxville: University of Tennessee Press, 1987), chapter 7; David McBride, *From TB to AIDS: Epidemics Among Urban Blacks since 1900* (Albany: State University of New York Press, 1991), chapter 4.

2. Raymond Wolters, *Negroes and the Great Depression: The Problem of Economic Recovery* (Westport, Conn.: Greenwood Press, 1970); Harvard Sitkoff, *A New Deal for Blacks: The Emergence of Civil Rights as a National Issue* (New York: Oxford University Press, 1978); Edward H. Beardsley, "Race as a Factor in Health," in *Women, Health and Medicine in America: A Historical Handbook*, ed. Rima D. Apple (New York: Garland, 1990), 121–40.

3. George Rosen, *A History of Public Health* (New York: MD Publications, 1958), 382.

4. After years of exhaustive searching, with assistance from Aloha South of the National Archives and Peter Hirtle of the National Library of Medicine, I was never able to locate the records of the Office of Negro Health Work at the Public Health Service or the personal papers of Dr. Roscoe C. Brown. All indications suggest that they are no longer available. Dr. Roscoe Brown Jr., son of the late Dr. Brown and president of Bronx City College, remembered that the family donated his father's papers to Howard University in the early 1960s, but archivists of Moorland-Spingarn Research Center, Howard University, Washington, D.C., were unable to locate them or any records of deposit.

5. "Negro Health," *Time*, 8 April 1940, 41.

6. [Dr. Montague Cobb], "National Negro Health Program Ends," *Journal of the National Medical Association* 43 (May 1951): 199; and "Dr. Roscoe C. Brown Receives High Federal Awards," *Journal of the National Medical Association* 44 (March 1952): 151–52.

7. Brown was an editor of the dental section of the *Journal of the National Medical Association* during the 1910s, a founder of the Old Dominion State Dental Society of Virginia in 1913, and one of the eighteen trustees to sign the certificate of incorporation for the NMA in 1923. John A. Kenney, *The Negro in Medicine* (n.p.: John A. Kenney, 1912), 31; G. James Fleming and Christian E. Burckel, eds., *Who's Who in Colored America*, 7th ed. (Yonkers-on-Hudson, New York: Christian E. Burckel & Associates, 1950), 88; Clifton O. Dummett, and Lois Doyle Dummett, *Afro-Americans in Dentistry: Sequence and Consequence of Events* (n.p.: Clifton Dummett, 1978), 20, 22, 26–27.

8. "Dr. Roscoe C. Brown Receives High Federal Awards"; Memorandum, Negro Health Week Planning Meeting, Washington, D.C., 30 October 1928, and Proceedings of the Negro Health Week Planning Meeting, Washington, D.C., 19 October 1929, file cabinet 3, drawer 1, Department of Records and Research Collection, Hollis Burke Frissell Library, Tuskegee University, Tuskegee, Ala.

9. "Employees of the Division of Venereal Diseases," 16 January 1922, box 165, general records, Division of Venereal Diseases, 1918–1936, Record Group 90, United States Public Health Service (USPHS), National Archives, Washington, D.C.; W. C. Blassingame to R. B. Stewart, 10 May 1922, and Thomas Campbell to J. A. Evans, 11 May 1922, Correspondence 1922, box 101, Record Group 33, U.S. Extension Service, National Archives, Washington, D.C.; *Annual Report of the Surgeon General of the Public Health Service of the United States for the fiscal year 1919* [hereinafter *Annual Report of the USPHS*] (Washington, D.C.: U.S. Government Printing Office, 1919), 281, 297; *Annual Report of the USPHS* (1920), 337; *Annual Report of the USPHS* (1923), 268; *Annual Report of the USPHS* (1924), 244.

10. C. C. Pierce, Proceedings of the Negro Health Week Planning Meeting, 1 November 1926, file cabinet 3, drawer 1, Department of Records and Research Collection.

11. Roscoe Brown to Robert Moton, 2 January 1922, and Brown to Moton, 8 February 1923, box 80, general correspondence, Robert Russa Moton Papers, Hollis Burke Frissell Library, Tuskegee University, Tuskegee, Ala.; C. C. Pierce, Proceedings of the Negro Health Week Planning Meeting, Washington, D.C., 29 October 1930, file cabinet 3, drawer 2, Department of Records and Research Collection.

12. Roscoe C. Brown to Robert Moton, 26 March 1923; C. C. Pierce, Acting Surgeon General, to Roscoe Brown, 26 March 1927; Roscoe Brown to Assistant Surgeon General Thomas Parran, 16 April 1927, box 174, general records, Division of Venereal Diseases, 1918–1936, Record Group 90, USPHS.

13. Mary Gover, "Mortality Among Negroes in the United States," Public Health Bulletin 174 (Washington, D.C.: U.S. Government Printing Office, 1928). Brown had requested a study of morbidity and mortality but was pleased that at least something was done. Roscoe Brown to Surgeon General Cumming, 20 February 1926, and Cumming to Brown 2 March 1926, and Brown to Cumming, 8 March 1926, box 197, general records, 1924–1935, Record Group 90, USPHS; Roscoe C. Brown, "An Open Letter to Those Interested in the Health of the Negro in This County," *National Notes* 30 (May 1928): 18.

14. Judith Walzer Leavitt, *The Healthiest City: Milwaukee and the Politics of Health Reform* (Princeton, N.J.: Princeton University Press, 1982), 200–201, 204; Beardsley, *A History of Neglect*, 98.

15. The gender of these black physicians is unspecified, but I think it is safe to assume that they are speaking of men. See Todd L. Savitt, "Entering A White Profession: Black Physicians in the New South," *Bulletin of the History of Medicine* 61 (Winter 1987): 507–40; Beardsley, *A History of Neglect*, chapter 4.

16. Carl G. Robert, National Medical Association Presidential Address, 1927, box 19, Louis T. Wright Papers, Manuscript Division, Moorland-Spingarn Research Center, Howard University, Washington, D.C.

17. Dr. T. Spotuas Burwell to Robert Moton, 3 December 1928, box 156,

general correspondence, Moton Papers; Dr. D. W. Byrd to Emmett J. Scott, 7 July 1917, box 7, local correspondence, Moton Papers.

18. Herbert M. Morais, *The History of the Negro in Medicine* (New York: Publishers Company for the Association for the Study of Negro Life and History, 1967), 100.

19. W. O. Saunders, "Gold Tooth," in *These Are Our Lives*, by the Federal Writers' Project (Chapel Hill: University of North Carolina Press, 1939, copyright renewed 1967; reprint W. W. Norton, 1975), 295.

20. Dr. Boothe to Booker T. Washington, 15 April 1915, microfilm reel 379, general correspondence, Booker T. Washington Papers, Library of Congress, Washington, D.C.

21. Louisville, Ky., Health Week Report, 1927, submitted by Mary L. Hicks, Secretary of the Kentucky Inter-racial Commission, box 132, general correspondence, Moton Papers.

22. Wiley A. Hall, Executive Secretary of the Richmond Urban League, to Monroe Work, 13 May 1930; Richmond Health Week Report, 1930, file cabinet 2, drawer 2, Department of Records and Research Collection.

23. For descriptions of health week events see *Howard Medical News*, 20 March 1927; *Howard Medical News* 20 March 1928; *Howard Medical News* 20 May 1928; *Journal of the National Medical Association* 9 (July–September 1917): 142; C. C. Jones to Albon Holsey, 15 February 1929, file cabinet 3, drawer 1, Department of Records and Research Collection.

24. Dr. Bousfield to Dr. C. C. Cater of Atlanta Life Insurance Company, 27 March 1933, box 4, Series C, Correspondence, Peter Marshall Murray Papers, Manuscript Division, Moorland-Spingarn Research Center, Howard University, Washington, D.C.

25. Paul Starr, *The Social Transformation of American Medicine* (New York: Basic Books, 1982), 193.

26. Algernon B. Jackson to Booker T. Washington, 11 January 1915, microfilm reel 382, general correspondence, Washington Papers.

27. *Negro Health Week Bulletin* for 1927, 1928, and 1929, located in government documents, Wisconsin State Historical Society Library, Madison, Wis.

28. They were Dr. George W. Bowles, who had a private practice in Pennsylvania; Dr. Numa P. G. Adams, who in 1929 became the first black dean of Howard University Medical School; Dr. Midian Othello Bousfield. Proceedings of the Negro Health Week Planning Meeting, 29 October 1930; W. Montague Cobb, "Numa P. G. Adams, M.D., 1885–1940," *Journal of the National Medical Association* 43 (January 1951): 43–52; "Dr. George Williams Bowles," *Journal of the National Medical Association* 44 (January 1952): 69–70; Peter Marshall Murray, M.D., "Midian O. Bousfield, M.D., 1885–1948," *Journal of the National Medical Association* 40 (May 1948): 120.

29. Roscoe C. Brown, Minutes of Executive Committee, 19 January 1932, file cabinet 3, drawer 3, Department of Records and Research Collection; radio broadcast by Dr. Felix J. Underwood, "Public Health and the Mississippi Negro," 7 April 1943, box 356, Record Group 51-Mississippi Department of Health, Mississippi Department of Archives and History, Jackson, Miss.; radio broadcast by Roscoe C.

Brown, "The Health Problem of the American Negro" 15 March 1932, box 199, general records 1924–1935, Record Group 90, USPHS; Minutes for the Subcommittee on Negro Health, Washington D.C., 17 December 1940, box 91, general classified files, Office of the Administration of the Federal Security Agency, Record Group 235, Department of Health, Education and Welfare (HEW), National Archives, Washington, D.C.

30. Roscoe C. Brown, Minutes of Executive Committee, 19 January 1932.

31. Proceedings of Negro Health Week conferences from 1926 to 1941, especially Proceedings of the Negro Health Week Planning Meeting, Washington, D.C., 1928; *National Negro Health News*, 1935 to 1945. On Mabel Keaton Staupers, see Darlene Clark Hine, "Mabel K. Staupers and the Integration of Black Nurses into the Armed Forces," in *Women and Health in America: Historical Readings*, ed. Judith Walzer Leavitt (Madison: University of Wisconsin Press, 1984), 497–506; on Modjeska Simpkins, see Beardsley, *A History of Neglect*, 108–12.

32. Roscoe C. Brown, Minutes of Executive Committee, 17 March 1931, file cabinet 3, drawer 2, Department of Records and Research Collection.

33. Roscoe C. Brown, "Program for the National Negro Health Movement" (1931), box 13, Murray Papers.

34. Roscoe C. Brown to Robert Moton, 31 December 1929, box 156, general correspondence, Moton Papers; Surgeon General Cumming to Robert Moton, 2 January 1930, and Acting Surgeon General Pierce to Monroe Work, 18 February 1930, file cabinet 3, drawer 1, Department of Records and Research Collection; Michael M. Davis of Rosenwald Fund to Dr. Numa Adams, 7 April 1931, file cabinet 3, drawer 2, Department of Records and Research Collection; Edwin R. Embree, *Annual Report of the Julius Rosenwald Fund* (1931), box 356, Record Group 51, Mississippi Department of Health.

35. Roscoe Brown to Robert Moton, 21 October 1929, file cabinet 3, drawer 1, Department of Records and Research Collection.

36. Will W. Alexander to C. C. Pierce, Acting Surgeon General, 8 October 1929, box 156, general correspondence, Moton Papers.

37. C. A. Lanon to Robert Moton, 9 November 1929, file cabinet 3, drawer 2, Department of Records and Research Collection.

38. G. E. Cannon to Surgeon General Blue, 2 March 1917, box 197, general records, 1924–1935, Record Group 90, USPHS.

39. Brown spent most of his career under Dr. Hugh Cumming, who was surgeon general from 1920 to 1936, and Dr. Thomas Parran, who held the position from 1936 to 1948. Bess Furman, *A Profile of the United States Public Health Service, 1798–1948* (Washington, D.C.: U.S. Government Printing Office, 1973), 389.

40. Roscoe Brown to Robert Moton, 3 September 1930, file cabinet 3, drawer 2, Department of Records and Research Collection. See also Assistant Surgeon General Pierce to Robert Moton, 3 September 1930, file cabinet 3, drawer 2, Department of Records and Research Collection.

41. Michael M. Davis to Robert Moton, 2 October 1930, file cabinet 3, drawer 2, Department of Records and Research Collection; Dr. Numa Adams to Monroe Work, 6 April 1932, box 58, local correspondence, Moton Papers; and [Dr. Midian Bousfield], "Recent Progress in the Program of the Julius Rosenwald Fund in

Negro Health" [1939?], box 599, Central File, 1937–1940, Record Group 102, Children's Bureau, National Archives, Washington, D.C.

42. [Bousfield], "Recent Progress in the Program of the Julius Rosenwald Fund in Negro Health"; W. Montague Cobb, "Fifty Years of Progress in Health," *Pittsburgh Courier* (1950), p. 6, located at Health Sciences Library, Howard University, Washington, D.C.

43. See correspondence in box 35, Central File, 1941–1944, Record Group 102, Children's Bureau; Dr. Martha M. Eliot to Rufus E. Clement, 11 January 1939, box 133, Correspondence and Reports, 1917–1954, Record Group 102, Children's Bureau; [Bousfield], "Recent Progress."

44. *Annual Report of the USPHS* (1933), 19; *Annual Report of the USPHS* (1938), 106; Dr. W. Montague Cobb, interview by the author, written notes, 26 July 1989, Washington, D.C.; Dr. Paul Cornely, interview by the author, tape recording, 24 July 1989, Howard University Medical School, Washington, D.C.; Mabel Keaton Staupers, interview by the author, tape recording, 30 July 1989, Washington, D.C.

45. *National Negro Health News* 12 (July–September 1944): back cover.

46. *Annual Report of the USPHS* (1943), 106.

47. Roscoe C. Brown, "The National Negro Health Week Movement," reprint from *Health Officer* 1 (September and October 1936): 146–51, 206–12. See also *National Negro Health News* from 1933 to 1950; Cornely, interview by the author.

48. Roscoe C. Brown to Robert Moton, 16 September 1932, box 58, local correspondence, Moton Papers.

49. *National Negro Health News* 4 (April–June 1936): 14; *National Negro Health News* 7 (July–September 1939): 22; *National Negro Health News* 8 (October–December 1940): 30.

50. *Annual Report of the USPHS* (1939), 106; *Annual Report of the USPHS* (1945), 24; *National Negro Health News* 13 (July–September 1945): 8.

51. Brown, "The National Negro Health Week Movement," 146–51, 206–12; "Negro Health Week Observance for the Six Years, 1925–1930," health week bulletin for 1931, file cabinet 3, drawer 2, Department of Records and Research Collection; annual reports of the USPHS for the 1930s and 1940s; *National Negro Health News* from 1933 to 1950.

52. Proceedings of the Negro Health Week Planning Meeting, 30 October 1928, file cabinet 3, drawer 1, Department of Records and Research Collection. See also Karen Buhler-Wilkerson, "False Dawn: The Rise and Decline of Public Health Nursing in America, 1900–1930," in *Nursing History: New Perspectives, New Possibilities*, ed. Ellen Condliffe Lagemann (New York: Teachers College Press, 1983), 89–106.

53. Monroe Work, "National Negro Health Week," *Public Health Nurse* 18 (March 1926): 120.

54. Barbara Melosh, *"The Physician's Hand": Work, Culture and Conflict in American Nursing* (Philadelphia: Temple University Press, 1982), chapter 4; Susan M. Reverby, *Ordered to Care: The Dilemma of American Nursing, 1850–1945* (Cambridge: Cambridge University Press, 1987), 109; Karen Buhler-Wilkerson, ed., *Nursing and the Public's Health: An Anthology of Sources* (New York: Garland, 1989);

Buhler-Wilkerson, "False Dawn"; Molly Ladd-Taylor, *Mother-Work: Women, Child Welfare, and the State, 1890–1930* (Urbana: University of Illinois Press, 1994), chapter 6.

55. Darlene Clark Hine, *Black Women in White: Racial Conflict and Cooperation in the Nursing Profession, 1890–1950* (Bloomington: Indiana University Press, 1989).

56. Morais, *The History of the Negro in Medicine*, 101.

57. Stanley Rayfield, Marjory Stimson, and Louise M. Tattershall, "A Study of Negro Public Health Nursing," *Public Health Nurse* 22 (October 1930): 525; Dr. Paul B. Cornely and M. S. Briscoe, "Public Health as a Professional Career," *Journal of the National Medical Association* 36 (May 1944): 77; "The 1946 Census of Public Health Nursing," *National Negro Health News* 14 (October–December 1946): 17; "Negro Public Health Nurses in the United States," *National Negro Health News* 6 (July–September 1938): 24–25; Philip and Beatrice Kalisch, *The Advance of American Nursing* (Boston: Little, Brown, 1978), 558; Hine, *Black Women in White*, 227 n. 26.

58. Emily W. Bennett, "The Work of a Rosenwald Nurse," *Public Health Nurse* 23 (March 1931): 119–20.

59. "Health Clubs for Negro Women," *National Negro Health News* 5 (October–December 1937): 16.

60. Pearl McIver, "Rural Nursing," *Journal of the National Medical Association* 28 (May 1936): 87.

61. McIver, "Rural Nursing," 87–89.

62. Memo from Roscoe Brown to Robert Olesen, 2 September 1936, box 195, general files 1936–1944, Record Group 90, USPHS; "The Negro Nurse in 17 Agencies," *Public Health Nurse* 33 (1941): 463; Anne Arundel County, Maryland, Health Week Report, 1930, file cabinet 3, drawer 2, Department of Records and Research Collection.

63. *National Negro Health News* 8 (July–September 1940): 31.

64. Cardinal Gibbons Institute, Saint Mary's County, Md., Health Week Report, 1930, submitted by Victor H. Daniel, Chairman, and Constance E. H. Daniel, Secretary, to Tuskegee Institute, 21 April 1930, file cabinet 3, drawer 2, Department of Records and Research Collection.

65. Cardinal Gibbons Institute Health Week Report.

66. Dr. R. H. Riley, Director of the Maryland Department of Health, to Robert Moton, 13 May 1930, and Wicomico County, Md., Health Week Report, 1930, submitted by Seth H. Hurdle, M.D., County Health Officer for Wicomico County, file cabinet 3, drawer 2, Department of Records and Research Collection.

67. Dr. M. V. Hargett, Director of East Carroll Parish Health Unit, 3 May 1930. See also East Carroll Parish, La., Health Week Report, 1930, file cabinet 3, drawer 2, Department of Records and Research Collection.

68. Elizabeth White Tipton, "Sure Progress in Montgomery County, Maryland," *National Negro Health News* 16 (July–September 1948): 10; "How to Form a Health Council," *National Negro Health News* 16 (July–September 1948): 11–12.

69. Editorial, "Health Week 1915–1944," *Philadelphia Afro-American*, 8 April 1944, p. 5.

70. Elizabeth Fee, "Sin vs. Science: Venereal Disease in Baltimore in the Twen-

tieth Century," *Journal of the History of Medicine and Allied Sciences* 43 (April 1988): 141–64, especially 145, 148, 154.

71. Walter White to President Harry S Truman, 21 October 1947, box 25, general records, Office of the Administrator, alphabetical series, 1944–1950, Record Group 235, HEW.

72. [Dr. John Kenney?], "Recognition of the Negro Medical Profession in Public Health Work," *Journal of the National Medical Profession* 27 (February 1935): 29.

73. Morais, *The History of the Negro in Medicine*, chapters 8 and 9; Beardsley, *A History of Neglect*, chapter 11; Walter White to Peter Marshall Murray, 16 June 1932, box 6, Series C, Correspondence, Murray Papers.

74. White to President Truman, 21 October 1947.

75. Affidavit by Pearl Miles, box 15, Records of the National Council of Negro Women, Series 5, Subject Files, 1942–1949, Bethune Museum and Archives, Washington, D.C.

76. For background on the National Council of Negro Women, see Dr. Bettye Collier-Thomas, *N.C.N.W., 1935–1980* (Washington, D.C.: National Council of Negro Women, 1981).

77. Cornely, interview by the author. For a discussion of a similar pattern among whites in rural areas, see Frederick D. Mott and Milton I. Roemer, *Rural Health and Medical Care* (New York: McGraw-Hill, 1948), 468.

78. *National Negro Health News* 11 (April–June 1943), inside cover. See also Whitney M. Young Jr., Executive Director of the National Urban League, "The Role of the Middle-Class Negro," *Ebony* 18 (September 1963): 67–71.

79. [Roscoe C. Brown], "Fact Sheet for the 1949 National Negro Health Week," box 356, Record Group 51, Mississippi Department of Health.

80. Quote from Brown in [Dr. Montague Cobb], "National Negro Health News Ceases Publication," *Journal of the National Medical Association* 43 (January 1951): 59.

81. Dr. W. Montague Cobb, "National Negro Health Program Ends," 198–99.

82. [Roscoe C. Brown], *National Negro Health News* 18 (April–June 1950): 1. See also "National Negro Health Week," *American Journal of Public Health* 40 (February 1950): 240.

83. [Roscoe C. Brown], "The National Negro Health Week Movement," *National Negro Health News* 18 (April–June 1950): 2.

84. [Brown], "The National Negro Health Week Movement," 2.

85. 1950 National Negro Health Week announcement. See also "Fact Sheet," box 356, Record Group 51, Mississippi Department of Health.

86. Jessie Parkhurst Guzman, ed., *The Negro Year Book, 1952: A Review of Events Affecting Negro Life* (New York: William H. Wise, 1952), 169; Roscoe Brown to Mary McLeod Bethune, 10 October 1949, Records of the National Council of Negro Women, Series 5, subject files, box 5; and [Montague Cobb], "National Negro Health Program Ends," 199.

87. "Dr. Roscoe C. Brown Receives High Federal Awards," 151–152; "Dr. Roscoe C. Brown Retires from Public Health Service," *Journal of the National Medical Association* 47 (July 1955): 274, 283; poem by Dr. Roscoe C. Brown, "At Seventy-

Five," reprinted from *The Dragon* (November 1959) (courtesy of Dr. Roscoe C. Brown, Jr.); "Brown, Roscoe Conkling," *Washington Post-Herald*, 28 October 1954, Vertical File, Moorland-Spingarn Research Center Library, Howard University; Roscoe C. Brown, Jr., telephone interview by the author, 29 September 1988.

88. Cobb, "Fifty Years of Progress in Health," 4; Cobb, interview by the author.

89. [Cobb], "National Negro Health News Ceases Publication," 59.

90. Cobb, "Numa P. G. Adams, M.D., 1885–1940," 48.

91. Louis T. Wright, autobiographical manuscript, n.d., box 1, Wright Papers.

92. Louis T. Wright, "Health Problems of the Negro," *Interracial Review* (January 1935), p. 7, box 6, Wright Papers; [Montague Cobb?], "Louis T. Wright, M.D.," *Journal of the National Medical Association* 30 (August 1937): 112–13.

93. "Dr. Wright Socks Health Week in the Eye," *Philadelphia Afro-American*, 26 March 1938, p. 13

94. Joint statement by Wright and Hill, 1938 National Health Conference, Washington, D.C., box 6, Wright Papers.

95. Louis T. Wright, "Report on the Health of the Negro" (1952), box 6, Wright Papers.

96. Cornely, interview by the author. For biographical information on Cornely, see Hildrus Poindexter, *My World of Reality* (Detroit: Balamp Publishing, 1973), 119; Beardsley, *A History of Neglect*, 93–94, 261–263; Morais, *The History of the Negro in Medicine*, 100, 130.

97. Cornely, interview by the author; Cobb, interview by the author; Poindexter, *My World of Reality*, 170.

98. By 1935 there were 45 African Americans working for Roosevelt in federal departments and New Deal agencies. Sitkoff, *A New Deal for Blacks*, 78, 80. See also Alvin White, "What Has Become of the New Dealers?" *Philadelphia Afro-American*, 5 April 1947, p. M-4.

99. Wiley A. Hall, Executive Secretary of Richmond Urban League, to Monroe Work, 13 May 1930. See also Richmond Health Week Report, 1930, Department of Records and Research Collection.

Chapter 4

1. M. M. Hubert to Thomas Campbell, 26 May 1922, box 101, Correspondence 1922, Record Group 33, U.S. Extension Service, National Archives, Washington, D.C. On the history of the school, see B. D. Mayberry, "The Role of Tuskegee University in the Origin, Growth and Development of the Negro Extension Service," unpublished manuscript (1988), p. 111 (author's possession); Thomas Monroe Campbell, *The Movable School Goes to the Negro Farmer* (Tuskegee, Ala.: Tuskegee Institute Press, 1936; reprint, New York: Arno Press and the New York Times, 1969), 145.

2. James H. Jones, *Bad Blood: The Tuskegee Syphilis Experiment* (New York: Free Press, 1981; expanded edition 1993), 91 (page numbers refer to the 1981 edition).

3. Eunice Rivers Laurie, interview by A. Lillian Thompson, 10 October 1977, Black Women Oral History Project, from the Arthur and Elizabeth Schlesinger Library on the History of Women in America, Radcliffe College, Cambridge, Mass. Published in Ruth Edmonds Hill, ed., *The Black Women Oral History Project*, vol. 7 (Westport, Conn.: Meckler, 1991), 213–42. See also J. Jones, *Bad Blood*, 6, 158; Allan Brandt, "Racism and Research: The Case of the Tuskegee Syphilis Study," in *Sickness and Health in America: Readings in the History of Medicine and Public Health*, ed. Judith Walzer Leavitt and Ronald L. Numbers (Madison: University of Wisconsin Press, 1984), 331–43, especially 337; Darlene Clark Hine, *Black Women in White: Racial Conflict and Cooperation in the Nursing Profession, 1890–1950* (Bloomington: Indiana University Press, 1989), 154–56.

4. Louis Harlan, *Booker T. Washington: The Wizard of Tuskegee, 1901–1915* (New York: Oxford University Press, 1983), chapter 9.

5. Manning Marable, "The Politics of Black Land Tenure, 1877–1915," *Agricultural History* 53 (January 1979): 144.

6. Monroe Work, "Racial Factors and Economic Forces in Land Tenure in the South," *Social Forces* 15 (December 1936): 214–15 (located in box 11, Monroe Nathan Work Papers, Hollis Burke Frissell Library, Tuskegee University, Tuskegee, Ala.); Charles S. Johnson, *Shadow of the Plantation* (Chicago: University of Chicago Press, 1934), 7, 104, 109, 112, 128; Marable, "The Politics of Black Land Tenure," 144; and Pete Daniel, *Standing at the Crossroads: Southern Life Since 1900* (New York: Hill and Wang, 1986), 7.

7. Campbell, *The Movable School*, 80–81.

8. T. J. Woofter, "Organization of Rural Negroes For Public Health Work," *National Conference of Social Work Proceedings*, fiftieth session (1923): 74.

9. M. M. Hubert to Thomas Campbell, 26 May 1922; Thomas Campbell to P. K. Yonge, 6 June 1922, Correspondence 1922, box 101, Record Group 33, U.S. Extension Service; Campbell, *The Movable School*, 92–93, 145; Mayberry, "The Role of Tuskegee University," 111; Allen W. Jones, "The South's First Black Farm Agents," *Agricultural History* 50 (October 1976): 636–44; Harlan, *Booker T. Washington: Wizard*, 208.

10. *Proceedings of Session on Negro Social Work at the Alabama Conference of Social Work*, 9 April 1929, p. 15 (located in box 1, Work Papers); Campbell, *The Movable School*, 81, 93; Earl W. Crosby, "Limited Success Against Long Odds: The Black County Agent," *Agricultural History* 57 (July 1983): 281; Joel Schor, "The Black Presence in the U.S. Cooperative Extension Service Since 1945: An American Quest for Service and Equity," *Agricultural History* 60 (Spring 1986): 139.

11. Crosby, "Limited Success," 281 n.5; statement, 14 March 1925, Correspondence 1909–1923, Negroes, box 2, Record Group 16, Office of the Secretary of Agriculture, National Archives, Washington, D.C.; A. Jones, "The South's First Black Farm Agents," 643; Mayberry, "The Role of Tuskegee University," 39; Debra Newman, *Black History: A Guide to Civilian Records in the National Archives* (Washington, D.C.: National Archives Trust Fund Board, 1984), 22; Gladys L. Baker, *The County Agent* (Chicago: University of Chicago Press, 1939), 197.

12. Edward R. Lloyd, Director of Extension in Mississippi to Washington, D.C., 21 May 1918, Correspondence 1918, box 26. See also L. N. Duncan to O. B.

Martin, 1 October 1913, Correspondence 1914, Alabama, box 4, Record Group 33, U.S. Extension Service.

13. Robert Moton to Secretary of Agriculture Henry Wallace, 22 March 1921, Correspondence 1909–1923, Negroes, box 1, Record Group 16, Office of the Secretary of Agriculture; Harry Sims, "Striking Example of How the Rural Home Problems Are Being Solved by Movable School," *Rural Messenger* 1 (December 1920): 2; "Tuskegee's Schools on Wheels," *Durant's Standard* 1 (August 1923): 11–12; A. Florence May, "Education Carried to the Door of the Farmer," *Tuskegeean* (August–September 1931): 28; Campbell, *The Movable School*, 82, 91; Harlan, *Booker T. Washington: Wizard*, 207–8.

14. Summary Report of Tuskegee Movable School, October 1922, Correspondence 1909–1923, Negroes, box 1, Record Group 16, Office of the Secretary of Agriculture; "Tuskegee's Schools On Wheels"; Campbell, *The Movable School*, 109, 120–21.

15. John M. Gaus and Leon O. Wolcott, *Public Administration and the United States Department of Agriculture* (Chicago: 1940; reprint, New York: Da Capo Press, 1975), 19.

16. Campbell, *The Movable School*, 118, 121, 126; Correspondence 1916–1917, Alabama, box 12, Record Group 33, U.S. Extension Service; Allen W. Jones, "Thomas M. Campbell: Black Agricultural Leader of the New South," *Agricultural History* 53 (January 1979): 45; Marable, "The Politics of Black Land Tenure," 150.

17. Campbell, *U.S. Farm Demonstration Work Among Negroes in the South*, 22 February 1915, p. 3, box 989, Booker T. Washington Papers, Library of Congress, Washington, D.C. See also Campbell, *The Movable School*, part 1, chapter 1; A. Jones, "The South's First Black Farm Agents," 644.

18. Gaus and Wolcott, *Public Administration*, 228–30.

19. Monroe Work, "How Tuskegee Has Improved a Black Belt County" [1909?], pp. 25, 29–30, box 3, Work Papers.

20. William J. Breen, "Black Women and the Great War: Mobilization and Reform in the South," *Journal of Southern History* 44 (August 1978): 436–37. See also Joan M. Jensen, "Crossing Ethnic Barriers in the Southwest: Women's Agricultural Extension Education, 1914–1940," *Agricultural History* 60 (Spring 1986): 169–81.

21. *The Rural Messenger* 2 (May–June 1921): 6; *Southern Letter* 32 (August 1915): 4; "The Juanita Coleman Hospital," *Southern Letter* 40 (January 1924): 4; A. Jones, "Thomas M. Campbell," 47; Campbell, *The Movable School*, 106.

22. L. R. Daly, Report for Macon County, 1930, p. 9, Extension Agents Reports, microfilm reel 58, Record Group 33, U.S. Extension Service; Correspondence 1916–1917, Alabama, box 12, Record Group 33, U.S. Extension Service; Campbell, *The Movable School*, 109, 121, 126, 128–30; Alice C. Oliver, "Home Demonstration Work in Mississippi," *Rural Messenger* 1 (April 1921): 1; Jessie M. Rodrique, "The Black Community and the Birth-Control Movement," in *Unequal Sisters: A Multicultural Reader in U.S. Women's History*, ed. Ellen Carol DuBois and Vicki L. Ruiz (New York: Routledge, 1990), 333–44, especially 340.

23. Report by C. W. Warburton, Director of Extension Work, to J. C. Leukhardt, Interdepartmental Committee on Health and Welfare Activities in the Trea-

sury Department, 1 June 1936, box 394, Record Group 33, U.S. Extension Service; Thomas Campbell, "Extension Work Among Negroes in the South," Correspondence 1935, box 290, Record Group 33, U.S. Extension Service; Proceedings of the Negro Health Week Planning Meeting, 1 November 1926, morning session, p. 10; Monroe R. Work, "National Negro Health Week," *Public Health Nurse* 18 (March 1926): 120; *Rural Messenger* 1 (26 May 1920): 9.

24. Campbell, "Extension Work."

25. Laura Daly, "The Approach of the Rural Welfare Worker to the Negro Family Welfare Problem," *Proceedings of Session on Negro Social Work*, 9 April 1929, p. 12.

26. Daly, *Proceedings*, 13–14. See also Onnie Lee Logan, *Motherwit: An Alabama Midwife's Story* (New York: E. P. Dutton, 1989), 19; Thordis Simonsen, ed., *You May Plow Here: The Narrative of Sara Brooks* (New York: Touchtone Books, Simon and Schuster, 1986), 137.

27. Daly, *Proceedings*, pp. 13–14.

28. L. C. Hanna, "Making A Fireless Cooker," *Proceedings of Session on Negro Social Work*, 9 April 1929, pp. 18–19.

29. Daly, *Proceedings*, pp. 13–14; Hanna, *Proceedings*, pp. 18–19.

30. Daly, *Proceedings*, p. 12; Campbell, "Extension Work."

31. Daly, *Proceedings*, pp. 13–14.

32. L. R. Daly, Report for Macon County, 1935, p. 7, Extension Agents Reports, microfilm reel 58, Record Group 33, U.S. Extension Service.

33. Campbell, *The Movable School*, 119, see also 93–94. See also Cynthia Neverdon-Morton, *Afro-American Women of the South and the Advancement of the Race, 1895–1925* (Knoxville: University of Tennessee Press, 1989), 33.

34. Campbell, *The Movable School*, 153–54. See also Campbell, *U.S. Farm Demonstration Work*; M. M. Hubert, "Extension Work in Mississippi Helps Negro Farmers," *Rural Messenger* 1 (July 1920): 4.

35. "Movable Schools for Negro Farmers," *Southern Letter* 32 (November 1915): 1; *Southern Letter* (January 1915): 3; Thomas Campbell, Report of Movable School Work, to J. F. Duggar, 2 October 1915, Correspondence 1915–16, box 8, Record Group 33, U.S. Extension Service; Correspondence 1918, Alabama, box 16, Record Group 33, U.S. Extension Service; Thomas Campbell, Report of Movable School Work, to Washington, D.C., August 1922, box, 6, Tuskegee Institute Extension Service Collection, Hollis Burke Frissell Library, Tuskegee University, Tuskegee, Ala.; Annual Report of the Movable School Work, 31 December 1928, box 50, Thomas Monroe Campbell Papers, Hollis Burke Frissell Library, Tuskegee University, Tuskegee, Ala.

36. Juanita Coleman, *Rural Messenger* 2 (July 1921): 10–11.

37. Campbell, *The Movable School*, 117–118, 125; "Tuskegee's Schools on Wheels."

38. Thomas Campbell, "Writer Tells of Demonstration Work Carried On Among Colored Farmers by U.S. Government," *Nashville Globe and Independent* (located in Correspondence 1935, Alabama, box 290, Record Group 33, U.S. Extension Service). See also Baker, *The County Agent*, 203.

39. Campbell, *The Movable School*, 118, 147. See also "Booker T. Washington

Agricultural School on Wheels Awakens a Stir Among Negro Farmers of the South," *Southern Letter* 41 (September 1925): 1–4; C. A. Patillo to G. W. Goodwin, 24 April 1922, in "Agricultural Extension Work Among Negroes in Alabama," Monthly Report of Movable School Work, April 1922, Correspondence 1909–1923, Negroes, box 1, Record Group 16, U.S. Office of the Secretary of Agriculture; Campbell, Report of Movable School Work, to J. F. Duggar, 2 October 1915.

40. Patillo, "Agricultural Extension Work."

41. *Rural Messenger* 2 (May–June 1921): 7; Campbell, *The Movable School*, 117; Correspondence 1916–1917, Alabama, box 12, Record Group 33, U.S. Extension Service; Annual Report of the Movable School Work, 31 December 1928.

42. Campbell, *The Movable School*, 98, see also 96–97.

43. Campbell, Report of Movable School Work, to J. F. Duggar, 2 October 1915. See also "Booker T. Washington Agricultural School on Wheels"; William J. Maddox, "Wheeled Schools Deliver Education," box 8, Tuskegee Institute Extension Service Collection; Annual Report of the Movable School Work, 31 December 1928.

44. Campbell, Report of Movable School Work, to J. F. Duggar, 2 October 1915.

45. Eunice Rivers, monthly reports of Movable School work for 1924, box 6, Tuskegee Institute Extension Service Collection. See also Monthly Report of Movable School Work, April 1922.

46. Monroe N. Work, "The South's Labor Problem," reprint from *South Atlantic Quarterly* 19 (January 1920): 7–8, located in finding aids folder, Work Papers. See also Pete Daniel, *The Shadow of Slavery: Peonage in the South, 1901–1969* (Urbana: University of Illinois Press, 1972, 1990); Daniel, *Standing at the Crossroads*, 54–58.

47. Campbell, *U.S. Farm Demonstration Work*, 6; Campbell, "Writer Tells of Demonstration Work"; A. Jones, "The South's First Black Farm Agents," 642.

48. Daly, Proceedings of the Negro Health Week Planning Meeting, Tuskegee Institute, 20 January 1927, box 18, Campbell Papers.

49. Campbell, *U.S. Farm Demonstration Work*, 5.

50. Daniel, *The Shadow of Slavery*, 24, 30, 36, 139.

51. Campbell, *U.S. Farm Demonstration Work*, 6.

52. J. F. Drake, "How Whites and Negroes May Cooperate in Social Work for Negroes," *Proceedings of Session on Negro Social Work at the Alabama Conference of Social Work*, p. 7.

53. "Tuskegee's Schools on Wheels."

54. Johnson, *Shadow of the Plantation*, 25. See also Felix James, "The Tuskegee Institute Movable School, 1906–1923," *Agricultural History* 45 (July 1971): 204.

55. Campbell, *The Movable School*, 149.

56. George F. King, "Some Phases of Health Conditions Among Rural Negroes," *Rural Messenger* 3 (October 1922): 1.

57. Marcus Garvey to Secretary of Agriculture Henry C. Wallace, 4 October 1923, Correspondence 1909–1923, Negroes, box 1, Record Group 16, Office of the Secretary of Agriculture; Lerone Bennett Jr., "The Ghost of Marcus Garvey," *Ebony* 15 (March 1960): 53–61; Lawrence W. Levine, "Marcus Garvey and the Politics of

Revitalization," in *Black Leaders in the Twentieth Century*, ed. John Hope Franklin and August Meier (Chicago: University of Illinois Press, 1982), 105–38; Robert A. Hill, ed., *Marcus Garvey: Life and Lessons* (Berkeley: University of California Press, 1987).

58. Office of the Secretary of Agriculture to L. N. Duncan, 5 February 1923, correspondence 1909–1923.

59. Work, "The South's Labor Problem," 157; Monroe N. Work, "Inter-racial Cooperation," *Southern Workman* 49 (April 1920): 156–60; Blanche A. Beatty, "Negro Child Life in Rural Communities," *National Conference of Social Work Proceedings* (1924): 173–175; A. Jones, "Thomas M. Campbell," 49.

60. Campbell, *U.S. Farm Demonstration Work*, 3–4, 7. See also Campbell to C. B. Smith, 17 May 1922, Correspondence 1922, box 101, Record Group 33, U.S. Extension Service; Campbell, *The Movable School*, 153–54.

61. Campbell, *The Movable School*, 110, 153.

62. Eugene Tucker, *Helping Negroes to Become Better Farmers and Homemakers* (Washington, D.C.: U.S. Extension Service, 1921), a two-reel silent film, Accession 1431, Record Group 33.156 Extension Service, Motion Picture Reference Room, National Archives. For contemporary descriptions of the film, see *Rural Messenger* 2 (May–June 1921): 9; *Rural Messenger* 1 (August 1920): 6; and "Booker T. Washington Agricultural School on Wheels."

63. Baker, *The County Agent*, 200–203.

64. Daly, *Proceedings*, pp. 14–15.

65. Robert Moton to Miss Winifred C. Putnam, 10 November 1922, general correspondence, box 89, Robert Russa Moton Papers, Hollis Burke Frissell Library, Tuskegee University, Tuskegee, Ala.; Proceedings of the Negro Health Week Planning Meeting, 1 November 1926, afternoon session, p. 5; Molly Ladd-Taylor, *Raising a Baby the Government Way: Mothers' Letters to the Children's Bureau* (New Brunswick, N.J.: Rutgers University Press, 1986), 28.

66. Campbell, *The Movable School*, 111.

67. Campbell, *The Movable School*, 111–12.

68. Thomas Campbell, Proceedings of the Negro Health Week Planning Meeting, 1 November 1926.

69. *Rural Messenger* 1 (March 1921): 16; and Campbell, *The Movable School*, 122–23, 129, 131. See also Judith Walzer Leavitt, *The Healthiest City: Milwaukee and the Politics of Health Reform* (Princeton, N.J.: Princeton University Press, 1982), 222.

70. Uva M. Hester's report for her work in Montgomery County for the week of 19 June 1920 is reprinted in Campbell, *The Movable School*, 113–15.

71. Hester's report, reprinted in Campbell, *The Movable School*, 113.

72. *Rural Messenger* 1 (August 1920): 11.

73. Ibid.

74. Thomas Campbell to John Kenney, 27 January 1922; Campbell to Kenney, 21 February 1922; Campbell to Albon Holsey, 24 March 1922; Kenney to Campbell, 10 July 1922, box 6, Tuskegee Institute Extension Service Collection.

75. Monthly Report of Movable School Work, April 1922.

76. Eunice Rivers Laurie, interview, *The Black Women Oral History Project*, 220, 224; see also 216–19. See also Henry Howard, Report of Movable School,

1923, Extension agents reports, Alabama, microfilm reel 11, p. 2, Record Group 33, U.S. Extension Service; J. Jones, *Bad Blood*, 109–10; Hine, *Black Women in White*, 134, 154; Susan M. Reverby, "Laurie, Eunice Rivers (1899–1986)," in *Black Women in America: An Historical Encyclopedia*, ed. Darlene Clark Hine (New York: Carlson, 1993), 699–701.

77. Linda O. McMurry, *Recorder of the Black Experience: A Biography of Monroe Nathan Work* (Baton Rouge: Louisiana State University Press, 1985), 138.

78. Eunice Rivers, "Health Work with a Movable School," *Public Health Nurse* 18 (November 1926): 575–77; Eunice Rivers, reports on her Movable School work, monthly reports for 1924, box 6, Tuskegee Institute Extension Service Collection; Eunice Rivers Laurie, interview, *The Black Women Oral History Project*, 228; J. Jones, *Bad Blood*, 110; Hine, *Black Women in White*, 154.

79. Daly, Report for Macon County, 1930, microfilm reel 38, p. 9, Record Group 33, U.S. Extension Service. See also Johnson, *Shadow of the Plantation*, 197; Logan, *Motherwit*, 101–2.

80. *Proceedings of Session on Negro Social Work*, 9 April 1929, p. 15, box 1, Work Papers; Woofter, *Proceedings*, p. 72.

81. Letter from J. D. Barnes, "Serving the Community," printed in *Southern Letter* 45 (March–April 1929): 2.

82. Rivers, reports of Movable School work, monthly reports for 1924, box 6, Tuskegee Institute Extension Service Collection; Proceedings of the Negro Health Week Planning Meeting, 1 November 1926, afternoon session, p. 5; Rivers, "Health Work with a Movable School."

83. Eunice Rivers Laurie, interview, *The Black Women Oral History Project*, 234.

84. Eunice Rivers Laurie, interview, *The Black Women Oral History Project*, 230.

85. Rivers quoted in J. Jones, *Bad Blood*, 111.

86. *Annual Report of the Surgeon General of the Public Health Service of the United States for the fiscal year 1918* [hereafter *Annual Report of the USPHS*] (Washington, D.C.: Government Printing Office, 1918), 97; *Annual Report of the USPHS* (1919), 281 297; Allan M. Brandt, *No Magic Bullet: A Social History of Venereal Disease in the United States Since 1880* (New York: Oxford University Press, 1987), 56 77.

87. Paul Carley and O. C. Wenger, "The Prevalence of Syphilis in Apparently Healthy Negroes in Mississippi," *Journal of the American Medical Association* (7 June 1930) (located in box 356, Record Group 51, Mississippi Department of Health, Mississippi Department of Archives and History, Jackson, Miss.); *Annual Report of the USPHS* (1929), 273; "Recent Progress in the Program of the Julius Rosenwald Fund in Negro Health" [1938?], p. 9, Central File 1937–1940, box 599, Record Group 102, U.S. Children's Bureau, National Archives, Washington, D.C.; J. Jones, *Bad Blood*, 54, 59–60.

88. Louis T. Wright, "Factors Controlling Negro Health," *Crisis* 42 (September 1935): 264. See also J. Jones, *Bad Blood*, 23; Brandt, *No Magic Bullet*, 157–58; Brandt, "Racism and Research," 332; Elizabeth Fee, "Sin vs. Science: Venereal Disease in Baltimore in the Twentieth Century," *Journal of the History of Medicine and Allied Sciences* 43 (April 1988): 141–64.

89. Report to the Public Health Service by Dr. Vonderlehr, 10 July 1933, Division of Venereal Diseases, general records 1918–1936, box 182, Record Group 90, United States Public Health Service (USPHS), National Archives; J. Jones, *Bad Blood*, 27, 88, 92–95, 167. The development of Salvarsan in 1910, the first effective treatment for syphilis, prompted the end of the Oslo study. Brandt, *No Magic Bullet*, 40; and Brandt, "Racism and Research," 333–34. My thanks to Vanessa Northington Gamble for clarifying the ways in which the Oslo Study differed from the Tuskegee Syphilis Study.

90. Robert Moton to Hugh Cumming, 10 October 1932, general correspondence, box 180, Moton Papers; Eugene Dibble to Robert Moton, 17 September 1932, general correspondence, box 180, Moton Papers; J. Jones, *Bad Blood*, 74, 76.

91. Pete Daniel, "Black Power in the 1920s: The Case of Tuskegee Veterans Hospital," *Journal of Southern History* 36 (August 1970): 368–88; Vanessa Northington Gamble, "The Negro Hospital Renaissance: The Black Hospital Movement, 1920–1945," in *The American General Hospital: Communities and Social Contexts*, ed. Diana E. Long and Janet Golden (Ithaca, N.Y.: Cornell University Press, 1989), 101–2.

92. Roscoe C. Brown to W. Harry Barnes, president of the National Medical Association, 27 May 1936, and Roscoe C. Brown to Assistant Surgeon General Robert Olesen, 2 September 1936, Group 9, general records 1936–1944, box 195, Record Group 90, USPHS.

93. "Final Report of the National Medical Association Tuskegee Syphilis Study Ad Hoc Committee," 1 August 1973, p. 13, Moorland-Spingarn Research Center, Howard University, Washington, D.C.; J. Jones, *Bad Blood*, 7; Brandt, *No Magic Bullet*, 158.

94. Dr. Paul B. Cornely, interview by the author, tape recording, Howard University, Washington, D.C., 24 July 1989.

95. Shick, "Race, Class and Medicine," 104–5; J. Jones, *Bad Blood*, 167–68.

96. Eugene Dibble to Monroe Work, 9 September 1933, general correspondence, box 180, Moton Papers; *Annual Report of the USPHS* (1933), 96–97; J. Jones, *Bad Blood*, 68–69, 111, 114; Brandt, "Racism and Research," 335.

97. Quoted in Johnson, *Shadow of the Plantation*, 203.

98. J. Jones, *Bad Blood*, 104.

99. Vonderlehr, quoted in J. Jones, *Bad Blood*, 120.

100. Rivers, quoted in J. Jones, *Bad Blood*, 165.

101. J. Jones, *Bad Blood*, 68.

102. Quoted in J. Jones, *Bad Blood*, 80.

103. Eunice Rivers Laurie, interview, *The Black Women Oral History Project*, 232.

104. Eunice Rivers, Stanley H. Schuman, Lloyd Simpson, and Sidney Olansky, "Twenty Years of Followup Experience In a Long-Range Medical Study," *Public Health Reports* 68 (April 1953): 393; J. Jones, *Bad Blood*, 6, 69, 71, 73, 114; Brandt, "Racism and Research," 335 and 339; Hine, *Black Women in White*, 155–56.

105. J. Jones, *Bad Blood*, 163–64, 166; and Brandt, "Racism and Research," 337 n.

106. Rivers et al, "Twenty Years"; Rivers, "Health Work with a Movable School."

107. Rivers et al. "Twenty Years," 391–95; Catherine Corley, Department of Public Health, Alabama, to Eunice Rivers Laurie, Macon County Health Department, 26 May 1953, Eunice Rivers Laurie folder, Biographical Files, Hollis Burke Frissell Library, Tuskegee University, Ala.; J. Jones, *Bad Blood*, 161–62, 178.

108. Eunice Rivers Laurie, interview, *The Black Women Oral History Project*, 237. See also J. Jones, *Bad Blood*, 169.

109. J. Jones, *Bad Blood*, 128, 155, 160–61.

110. Thelma P. Walker, nomination letter for Eunice Rivers Laurie, 11 January 1972, Eunice Rivers Laurie folder, Biographical Files.

111. Eunice Rivers Laurie, interview, *The Black Women Oral History Project*, 231. See also J. Jones, *Bad Blood*, 107.

112. Brandt, "Racism and Research," 333. Furthermore, evidence suggests that not all the men had latent syphilis, given that when men in the control group (about 200 black men without syphilis) developed syphilis, the physicians merely switched them over to the untreated syphilitic group.

113. Eunice Rivers Laurie, interview, *The Black Women Oral History Project*, 229–30.

114. Eunice Rivers Laurie, interview, *The Black Women Oral History Project*, 232, 230–32. See also J. Jones, *Bad Blood*, 167.

115. Eunice Rivers Laurie, interview, *The Black Women Oral History Project*, 231.

116. Eunice Rivers Laurie, interview, *The Black Women Oral History Project*, 232.

117. J. Jones, *Bad Blood*, 164–65. Darlene Clark Hine found the explanations of James Jones "compelling" but suggested the possibility that Rivers "viewed the study as a way of ensuring for at least some blacks an unparalleled amount of medical attention." Hine, *Black Women in White*, 156.

118. J. Jones, *Bad Blood*, 97, 188–89; Jay Katz, *The Silent World of Doctor and Patient* (New York: Free Press, 1984), xvi, 1–4; David J. Rothman, *Strangers at the Bedside* (New York: Basic Books, 1991), 10, 47–48, 90, 247.

119. *Jet* [1973?], Eunice Rivers Laurie folder, Biographical Files, Tuskegee University.

Chapter 5

1. The major works on the history of lay midwifery include Frances K. Kobrin, "The American Midwife Controversy: A Crisis of Professionalization," *Sickness and Health in America: Readings in the History of Medicine and Public Health*, ed. Judith Walzer Leavitt and Ronald L. Numbers (Madison: University of Wisconsin Press, 1985), 197–205; Jane B. Donegan, *Women and Men Midwives: Medicine, Morality and Misogyny in Early America* (Westport, Conn.: Greenwood Press, 1978); Judy Barrett Litoff, *American Midwives, 1860 to the Present* (Westport, Conn.: Greenwood Press, 1978). See also Molly Ladd-Taylor, "'Grannies' and 'Spinsters': Midwife Education Under the Sheppard-Towner Act," *Journal of Social History* 22 (Winter 1988): 255–75; Charlotte G. Borst, "Catching Babies: The Change from

Midwife to Physician-Attended Childbirth in Wisconsin, 1870–1930" (Ph.D. diss., University of Wisconsin-Madison, 1989); Judy Litoff, "Midwives and History," in *Women, Health, and Medicine in America: A Historical Handbook*, ed. Rima D. Apple (New York: Garland, 1990), 443–58.

2. Southern midwives were most active in Mississippi, Alabama, Georgia, Florida, Louisiana, North Carolina, South Carolina, and Virginia. "Percentage of births attended by physicians and midwives and others, in certain states, as reported by State Bureaus of Child Hygiene for 1925," Central Files 1925–1928, box 274, Record Group 102, U.S. Children's Bureau, National Archives, Washington, D.C.; Elizabeth C. Tandy, "The Health Situation of Negro Mothers and Babies in the United States," Children's Bureau, March 1941, box 27, Record Group 51, Mississippi Department of Health, Mississippi Department of Archives and History, Jackson, Miss. Although this discussion focuses on black midwives in the Southeast, midwives in the Southwest faced similar historical patterns.

3. Mississippi State Board of Health, "Plan for the Division of Maternity and Infant Hygiene For 1922," Correspondence and Reports, 1917–1954, box 17, Record Group 102, Children's Bureau; Mississippi State Board of Health, "Study of Midwife Activities in Mississippi, July 1, 1921–June 30, 1929," 30 June 1929, box 36, Record Group 51, Mississippi Department of Health; and Mississippi State Board of Health, "The Relation of the Midwife to the State Board of Health," 1 July 1937, box 356, Record Group 51, Mississippi Department of Health.

4. Proceedings of the Negro Health Week Planning Meeting, Tuskegee, 20 January 1927, box 18, Thomas Monroe Campbell Papers, Hollis Burke Frissell Library, Tuskegee University, Tuskegee, Ala.; H. G. Perry, State Registrar of Vital Statistics, Alabama State Board of Health, to Jesse O. Thomas, 25 April 1921, and State Epidemiologist of North Carolina Board of Health to National Urban League, 12 May 1921, general office file, both in box A6, National Urban League Southern Regional Division, Library of Congress, Washington, D.C.; Emily Herring Wilson, *Hope and Dignity: Older Black Women of the South* (Philadelphia: Temple University Press, 1983), 39; Debra Anne Susie, *In the Way of Our Grandmothers: A Cultural View of Twentieth-Century Midwifery in Florida* (Athens: University of Georgia Press, 1988), 35; Edward H. Beardsley, *A History of Neglect: Health Care for Blacks and Mill Workers in the Twentieth-Century South* (Knoxville: University of Tennessee Press, 1987), 39.

5. See chart on white and black births in Mississippi, box 27, Record Group 51, Mississippi Department of Health; "The Relation of the Midwife to the State Board of Health," Mississippi State Board of Health, 1 January 1944, box 57, Record Group 51, Mississippi Department of Health; "History of Della Falkner: Mid-Wife and Register of Her Patients," published in Holly Springs, 26 February 1937, and newsclipping, "State Midwife Tells All In Booklet," 15 December 1937, box 27, Record Group 51, Mississippi Department of Health. See also Litoff, *American Midwives*, 27; Judy Barrett Litoff, *The American Midwife Debate: A Sourcebook on Its Modern Origins* (New York: Greenwood Press, 1986), 4; Tandy, "The Health Situation."

6. On black midwives see Molly C. Dougherty, "Southern Midwifery and Organized Health Care: Systems in Conflict," *Medical Anthropology: Cross Cultural*

Studies in Health and Illness 6 (Spring 1982): 113–26; Sharon A. Robinson, "A Historical Development of Midwifery in the Black Community: 1600–1940," *Journal of Nurse-Midwifery*, 29 (July/August 1984): 247–50; Linda Janet Holmes, "African American Midwives in the South," in *The American Way of Birth*, ed. Pamela S. Eakins (Philadelphia: Temple University Press, 1986), 273–91; Susie, *In the Way of Our Grandmothers*, viii, 16, 32; Onnie Lee Logan, *Motherwit: An Alabama Midwife's Story* (New York: E.P. Dutton, 1989); Ruth C. Schaffer, "The Health and Social Functions of Black Midwives on the Texas Brazos Bottom, 1920–1985," *Rural Sociology* 56 (Spring 1991): 89–105; Susan L. Smith, "White Nurses, Black Midwives, and Public Health in Mississippi, 1920–1950," *Nursing History Review* 2 (1994): 29–49.

7. Logan, *Motherwit*, 52, 58. See also Mrs. Jessie Guzman, interview by the author, tape recording, Tuskegee, Ala., 10 September 1989; Litoff, *American Midwives*, 28; Litoff, *The American Midwife Debate*, 4; "Report on the Midwife Survey in Texas," Bureau of Child Hygiene, Texas State Board of Health, 1924, Central File, 1925–1928, box 275, Record Group 102, Children's Bureau (reprinted in *The American Midwife Debate*, 67–81); Judith Walzer Leavitt, *Brought to Bed: Childbearing in America, 1750 to 1950* (New York: Oxford University Press, 1986), 108–9. Ruth C. Schaffer, in "The Health and Social Functions," states that the midwives in her study refused to provide cleaning assistance in order to disassociate themselves from black domestics (95).

8. Mississippi State Board of Health, "The Relation of the Midwife to the State Board of Health," 1 January 1935, box 2, Record Group 51, Mississippi Department of Health. Oral interviews and autobiographical accounts of midwives illustrate these points. See Logan, *Motherwit*; Susie, *In the Way of Our Grandmothers*, chapter 1; Linda Janet Holmes, "Thank You Jesus to Myself: The Life of a Traditional Black Midwife," in *The Black Women's Health Book: Speaking for Ourselves*, ed. Evelyn C. White (Seattle: Seal Press, 1990), 98–106; Mrs. Edna Roberts, interview by the author, tape recording, Mississippi, 17 September 1989. See also Laurel Thatcher Ulrich, *A Midwife's Tale: The Life of Martha Ballard, Based on Her Diary, 1785–1812* (New York: Knopf, 1990); Fran Leeper Buss, *La Partera: Story of A Midwife* (Ann Arbor: University of Michigan Press, 1980), 56–57.

9. Nurses Agnes B. Belser and Inez Driskell, "Report from Mary Osborne to Dr. Felix Underwood, Dr. Anna E. Rude, and Dr. W. S. Leathers," September 1923, Central File 1921–1924, box 248. See also excerpts from nurses in "Narrative and Statistical Report, June 1926," Correspondence and Reports 1917–1924, box 17, Record Group 102, Children's Bureau.

10. Nurse Louise James, Narrative and Statistical Report, November 1923, Mississippi State Board of Health, Central File, 1921–1924, box 249, Record Group 102, Children's Bureau.

11. See Borst, "Catching Babies," and Ulrich, *A Midwife's Tale*, 62.

12. See photographs of mothers and daughters in boxes 21 and 27; Mississippi State Board of Health, "The Relation of the Midwife to the State Board of Health," 1 January 1935; Brenda Boykin, "Midwives Recall Way Childbirth Used To Be," *Jackson Clarion-Ledger*, 15 February 1976; Beulah M. D'Olive Price, "'Birthin': A Past Life for an Alcorn Midwife," *Daily Corinthian*, 10 November 1976; Jack

Bleich, "Midwife's Delivery 82 Years Ago Began Tradition for Bessie Sutton," *Jackson Clarion-Ledger*, 17 November 1978, all in Midwives folder, Subject Files, Mississippi Department of Archives and History. See also Dougherty, "Southern Midwifery and Organized Health Care," 116; Susie, *In the Way of Our Grandmothers*, 10–13; Litoff, *American Midwives*, 32; Buss, *La Partera*, 34–35; Wilson, *Hope and Dignity*, 42; and Schaffer, "The Health and Social Functions," 94.

13. Thordis Simonsen, ed., *You May Plow Here: The Narrative of Sara Brooks* (New York: Touchtone Books, Simon and Schuster, 1986), 172. See also Litoff, *American Midwives*, 28; Ulrich, *A Midwife's Tale*, 197.

14. Bleich, "Midwife's Delivery." See also "Grannies: The Roots of Midwifery," *Jackson Clarion-Ledger*, 31 January 1982, Midwives folder, Subject Files, Mississippi Department of Archives and History; Wilson, *Hope and Dignity*, 43; Holmes, "African American Midwives in the South," 280–81; Logan, *Motherwit*, 103–4; Bernice Kelly Harris, "Plow Beams for Pills," in *These Are Our Lives* by the Federal Writers' Project (Chapel Hill: University of North Carolina Press, 1939, copyright renewed 1967; reprint W. W. Norton, 1975), 272; Schaffer, "The Health and Social Functions," 95.

15. "Leflore Mid-Wife Fails on Fee, Takes Baby," *Jackson Daily News*, 8 November 1939 (located in box 27, Record Group 51, Mississippi Department of Health). See also Price, "'Birthin': A Past Life"; Susie, *In the Way of Our Grandmothers*, 47.

16. Grace Abbott, Children's Bureau, to Governor Lee M. Russell, 12 December 1921, Central File 1921–1924, box 249, Record Group 102, Children's Bureau; "Plan for the Division of Maternity and Infant Hygiene For 1922." See also Joyce Antler and Daniel M. Fox, "The Movement Toward a Safe Maternity: Physician Accountability in New York City, 1915–1940," in *Sickness and Health in America*, ed. Leavitt and Numbers, 492; Litoff, *American Midwives*, 100; Molly Ladd-Taylor, *Raising a Baby the Government Way: Mothers' Letters to the Children's Bureau* (New Brunswick, N.J.: Rutgers University Press, 1986); Ladd-Taylor, "'Grannies' and 'Spinsters'"; Richard A. Meckel, *Save the Babies: American Public Health Reform and the Prevention of Infant Mortality, 1850–1929* (Baltimore: Johns Hopkins University Press, 1990), 210.

17. Litoff, *American Midwives*, 113; Barbara Melosh, *"The Physician's Hand": Work, Culture and Conflict in American Nursing* (Philadelphia: Temple University Press, 1982), 118; Logan *Motherwit*, introduction. Helpful discussions with Leslie Reagan facilitated my understanding of this important shift.

18. Dr. Felix Underwood, director of the Bureau of Child Welfare of the Mississippi State Board of Health, to Jesse O. Thomas, 3 May 1921, general office file, box A6, National Urban League Southern Regional Division Records.

19. Laurie Jean Reid, "The Plan of the Mississippi State Board of Health for the Supervision of Midwives," 1921 speech, box 354, Record Group 51, Mississippi Department of Health. See also Grace L. Meigs, U.S. Department of Labor, *Maternal Mortality from All Conditions Connected with Childbirth in the United States and Certain Other Countries*, Children's Bureau Publication No. 19 (Washington, D.C.: U.S. Government Printing Office, 1917); reprinted in Litoff, *The American Midwife Debate*, 50–66; and Litoff, *American Midwives*, 50–51, 55.

20. Leavitt, *Brought to Bed*, 271 (Glossary of Medical Terms).

21. Litoff, *The American Midwife Debate*, 5.

22. Lois Trabert, Bureau of Child Hygiene of Mississippi State Board of Health, to Dr. Anna E. Rude, Children's Bureau, 2 April 1923, Central File, 1921–1924, box 248, Record Group 102, Children's Bureau.

23. Mississippi State Board of Health, "Plan for the Division of Maternity and Infant Hygiene For 1922," "Study of Midwife Activities in Mississippi, July 1, 1921–June 30, 1929," "The Relation of the Midwife to the State Board of Health," 1 July 1937, and "The Relation of the Midwife to the State Board of Health," 1 January 1944. See also Neil R. McMillen, *Dark Journey: Black Mississippians in the Age of Jim Crow* (Urbana: University of Illinois Press, 1989), 169; Ulrich, *A Midwife's Tale*, 28.

24. Kobrin, "The American Midwife Controversy," 320; Litoff, *American Midwives*, 80; Litoff, *The American Midwife Debate*.

25. Nurse Agnes B. Belser, Narrative and Statistical Report, April 1924, Mississippi State Board of Health, Bureau of Child Hygiene and Public Health Nursing, Central File, 1921–1924, box 249, Record Group 102, Children's Bureau; Mississippi State Board of Health, "Midwife Activities in Mississippi" [1928?], State Boards of Health, Mississippi Cities and Counties, box 42, Record Group 90, United States Public Health Service (USPHS), National Archives, Washington, D.C.

26. Dr. F. J. Underwood, "The Development of Midwifery in Mississippi," read before the Southern Medical Association, 1925, box 36, Record Group 51, Mississippi Department of Health (also quoted in Litoff, *American Midwives*, 78).

27. Underwood's successor, Dr. Archie Lee Gray, was a staunch segregationist who served from 1958 to 1968. Biographical information on Underwood from folder, "Underwood, Felix Joel," Subject Files, and box 36, Record Group 51, Mississippi Department of Health; Lucie Robertson Bridgforth, "The Politics of Public Health Reform: Felix J. Underwood and the Mississippi State Board of Health, 1924–1958," *Public Historian* 6 (Summer 1984): 5–26.

28. Mary D. Osborne, "Public Health Nursing," 17 September 1938, box 317, Record Group 51, Mississippi Department of Health.

29. Roberts, interview by the author.

30. Roberts, interview by the author; "The Relation of the Midwife to the State Board of Health," 1 January 1935.

31. The first midwife manual in Mississippi was published in 1922. Lois Trabert, "Narrative Report of Work with Midwives, June 1921 to June 1922," Central File, 1921–1924, box 248, Record Group 102, Children's Bureau; Mississippi State Board of Health, *Manual for Midwives*, see 1928, 1939, and 1952 in box 354, and Mississippi State Board of Health, "Midwife Supervision" [1938?], box 36, all in Record Group 51, Mississippi Department of Health. Georgia first published a midwife manual in 1922, Florida in 1923. See Georgia State Board of Health, *Lessons for Midwives*, Child Hygiene Publication No. 17, Prenatal Series No. 3 [1922] (reprinted in Litoff, *The American Midwife Debate*, 200–207); Susie, *In the Way of Our Grandmothers*, 241 n.24.

32. Underwood, "The Development of Midwifery in Mississippi."

33. Photo entitled "A group of midwives in Madison County before any instructions," n.d., box 27, Record Group 51, Mississippi Department of Health; Ladd-Taylor, " 'Grannies' and 'Spinsters,' " 267.

34. Litoff, *American Midwives*, 101; Litoff, *The American Midwife Debate*, 10.

35. Dr. Felix J. Underwood, "Midwife Activities in Mississippi" [1932?], box 354; Mississippi State Board of Health, "The Relation of the Midwife to the State Board of Health," 1 July 1937; U.S. Bureau of the Census, reported in "The Relation of the Midwife to the State Board of Health" by the Mississippi State Board of Health," 27 April 1938, box 36; U.S. Bureau of the Census, reported in "The Relation of the Midwife to the State Board of Health" by the Mississippi State Board of Health, 1 January 1944, box 57, all in Record Group 51, Mississippi Department of Health. See also Antler and Fox, "The Movement Toward a Safe Maternity," 501; and Leavitt, *Brought to Bed*, 194.

36. Midwife club reports from the 1930s and 1940s, including Melissa Ann Mobley and J. E. Lucas, Carlisle Midwife Club, to Board of Health [1941?]; Midwife Report for Claiborne County, 9 August 1941; Irene B. Brisco and Louise Ceal, Humphreys County Midwife Club Report, 5 September 1942, all in box 27; photos of Coahoma County midwife meeting, 3 May 1951, box 21, Record Group 51, Mississippi Department of Health. See also Mary Osborne to Felix Underwood, "Narrative and Statistical Report, May 1924," Mississippi Bureau of Child Welfare and Public Health Nursing, Central File, 1921–1924, box 249, Record Group 102, Children's Bureau. See also Buss, *La Partera*, 53; and Susie, *In the Way of Our Grandmothers*, 46.

37. Silver nitrate was first used for newborns' eyes in the 1870s. This effort to prevent blindness was one of the only regulations mandated by the state legislature. Mississippi State Board of Health, "The Relation of the Midwife to the State Board of Health," 1 January 1935; Roberts, interview by the author; Litoff, *American Midwives*, 101; Litoff, *The American Midwife Debate*, 10; Susie, *In the Way of Our Grandmothers*, 4.

38. Violor Dorsy and Earline Morris, Hub, to Board of Health, box 36; photos of Holmes County midwife meeting, October 1938; and photos of Forrest County midwife meeting, n.d., in box 27, all in Record Group 51, Mississippi Department of Health. See also Dougherty, "Southern Midwifery and Organized Health Care," 116.

39. Lyrics to "Midwife Song: Protect the Mother and Baby" and "Song of the Midwives," sung to the tune of "As We Go Marching On," box 27; and Robert Loftus, "Stork Loses Two Long-Time Forrest County Helpers," *Hattiesburg American*, 29 November 1948, box 36, Record Group 51, Mississippi Department of Health.

40. John Lomax built a collection of black folk song recordings at the Library of Congress. *Mississippi Doctor*, 14 (June 1936–May 1937); and "Song's Recorder Here: Midwife Song Taken," newsclipping, 9 March 1937, box 36, Record Group 51, Mississippi Department of Health. See also article by Dr. James H. Ferguson, who described a visit to a midwife meeting in October 1948 at which a phonographic recording of the entire meeting was made. James H. Ferguson, "Mississippi Midwives," *Journal of the History of Medicine* (Winter 1950), 90–95, box 36, Record Group 51, Mississippi Department of Health.

41. Mississippi State Board of Health, "The Relation of the Midwife to the State Board of Health," 1 July 1937, box 356; "The Relation of the Midwife to the State Board of Health," 1 January 1944.

42. Ruth A. Dodd, "Midwife Supervision in South Carolina," *Public Health Nurse* (1920): 863 (courtesy of Leslie Schwalm). A nurse by the same name worked in Holmes County, Miss., in 1932. Ellen Woods Carter, Statistical Report, 1932, box 356, Record Group 51, Mississippi Department of Health.

43. Underwood, "The Development of Midwifery in Mississippi"; Mary Osborne to Dr. Haines, 10 November 1925, Central File, 1925–1928, box 330, Record Group 102, Children's Bureau.

44. Sallie Mae Brock and Virginia Thompson, Monroe County, *Examiner* (1944), box 36, Record Group 51, Mississippi Department of Health.

45. Dougherty, "Southern Midwifery and Organized Health Care," 117; Ladd-Taylor, "'Grannies' and 'Spinsters.'"

46. Reid, "The Plan of the Mississippi State Board of Health"; Litoff, *The American Midwife Debate*, 4; Holmes, "African American Midwives in the South," 286.

47. Quoted in Holmes, "African American Midwives in the South," 287.

48. Dr. W. E. Riecken, Jr., 17 July 1990, responses to written questions by author.

49. Nurse Elsie Davis, Holly Springs, "Nurses' Narrative Report, Mississippi State Board of Health, Bureau of Child Hygiene, Division of Public Health Nursing, July 1931," box 36, Record Group 51, Mississippi Department of Health.

50. Nurses Abbie G. Hall and Caroline Bourg, Sharkey-Issaquena Counties, "Nurses Narrative Report, Mississippi State Board of Health, Bureau of Child Hygiene, Division of Public Health Nursing, July 1931," box 36, Record Group 51, Mississippi Department of Health.

51. Otha Bell Jones, Itta Bena, to Board of Health, 13 April 1938, box 27, Record Group 51, Mississippi Department of Health. It was not unusual for midwives to keep excellent records of the births they delivered. Della Falkner kept a list of the name of every birth she attended for ten years from 1926 to 1936. "History of Della Falkner." See also Wilson, *Hope and Dignity*, 39.

52. Logan, *Motherwit*, 90. See also Ulrich, *A Midwife's Tale*, 181; Susie, *In the Way of Our Grandmothers*, 46.

53. Rosie Bell Rollins, West Point, to Lucy Massey, 13 November 1948, box 36, Record Group 51, Mississippi Department of Health.

54. Georgette Smith to the Supervisor of Midwives, 29 October 1945, box 27, Record Group 51, Mississippi Department of Health.

55. Quote from Nurse Mae Reeves in Mary Osborne report to Drs. Underwood, Rude, and Leathers.

56. Nurse report, Washington County, "Narrative and Statistical Report of the Mississippi Bureau of Child Welfare and Public Health Nursing," from Mary Osborne to Dr. Felix Underwood, May 1924, Central File, 1921–1924, box 249, Record Group 102, Children's Bureau.

57. Mrs. Zona C. Jelks, president, Mississippi Public Health Association, "My Twenty-Five Years in Public Health in Mississippi," talk at the annual conven-

tion, 29 November 1967, box 317, Record Group 51, Mississippi Department of Health.

58. Leslie J. Reagan, "When Abortion Was a Crime: The Legal and Medical Regulation of Abortion, Chicago, 1880–1973" (Ph.D. diss., University of Wisconsin-Madison, 1991), chapter 3. See also Leslie J. Reagan, "'About to Meet Her Maker': Women, Doctors, Dying Declarations, and the State's Investigation of Abortion, Chicago, 1867–1940," *Journal of American History* 77 (March 1991): 1240–64.

59. Ferguson, "Mississippi Midwives," 86.

60. Susie, *In the Way of Our Grandmothers*, 30.

61. Schaffer, "The Health and Social Functions," 96.

62. Logan, *Motherwit*, 115–17. Another method rural women used to induce miscarriage was drinking turpentine, according to a black woman from Alabama whose mother died from it. Simonsen, *You May Plow Here*, 160.

63. Susie, *In the Way of Our Grandmothers*, 30–31; Litoff, *American Midwives*, 30; Litoff, *The American Midwife Debate*, 8; Roberts, interview by the author.

64. Mississippi State Board of Health, "Midwife Supervision" [1938?]; Susan Tucker, *Telling Memories Among Southern Women: Domestic Workers and Their Employers in the Segregated South* (Baton Rouge: Louisiana State University Press, 1988), 177.

65. Mississippi State Board of Health, "Study of Midwife Activities in Mississippi, July 1, 1921–June 30, 1929"; Nurse Elois Conn, Amite County, *Southern Herald*, 12 November [1941?], box 27, Record Group 51, Mississippi Department of Health.

66. See Mississippi State Board of Health, *Manual for Midwives*, 1939; Nurse A. E. McDaniel, Tishomingo County, "Mississippi State Board of Health, Bureau of Child Hygiene and Public Health Nursing, Public Health Nurses' Narrative Reports," July 1928, box 41, Record Group 90, USPHS.

67. Underwood, "The Development of Midwifery in Mississippi"; Leavitt, *Brought to Bed*, 70.

68. Nurse Ethel B. Marsh, Adams County, "Nurses' Narrative Report, Mississippi State Board of Health, Bureau of Child Hygiene, Division of Public Health Nursing, July 1931," box 36, Record Group 51, Mississippi Department of Health.

69. Nurse Josie Strum, Clarke County, ibid.

70. Rose T. Coursey, Jones County, Welfare Worker, to Mary Osborne, 26 November 1927; Osborne's secretary to Coursey, 8 December 1933; Board of Health to Honorable Jack Deavours, County Attorney, 1 December 1933, box 36, Record Group 51, Mississippi Department of Health. Onnie Lee Logan in Alabama stated that she had a brother-in-law who was a midwife and had received a permit from the Board of Health. Logan, *Motherwit*, 30.

71. Quoted in "State Health Agency Calls Midwifery 'Dying Avocation,'" *Jackson Commercial Appeal* [1966?], box 36, Record Group 51, Mississippi Department of Health.

72. Dr. Felix J. Underwood, "Mary D. Osborne," *Mississippi Doctor* 24 (October 1946): 147–48 (located in box 354); Adda Osborne to Beatrice Butler, 31 July 1950, box 36, Record Group 51, Mississippi Department of Health. See also Edna

Roberts, "Biographical Sketch, Mary D. Osborne" (courtesy of Edna Roberts), author's possession; Roberts, interview by the author.

73. Bessie Ann Swearegan, midwife club leader, Torrance, to Mary Osborne, 1 August 1943, box 27, Record Group 51, Mississippi Department of Health. I have retained the spelling of the midwife letters, but added punctuation and capital letters at the start of sentences to ease reading.

74. See, for example, Lillie Bell Hill, "Annual Report For Lee County Midwife Club," 1937, box 27, Record Group 51, Mississippi Department of Health.

75. All letters are in box 36, Record Group 51, Mississippi Department of Health. My thanks to Leslie Schwalm for her helpful insights on the meanings of these letters.

76. Mary Cox, Tunica, to Massey, 23 July 1946, ibid.

77. Sarah Crosby, Puckett, to Lucy Massey, 22 July 1946, ibid.

78. Laura E. Scott, Lessley, to Lucy Massey, 26 July 1946, ibid. This phrase is also found in early nineteenth-century writings. See Ulrich, *A Midwife's Tale*, 253; Sterling, *We Are Your Sisters*, 102.

79. W. G. Crowley, Ruleville, to Lucy Massey, 16 August 1946, box 36, Record Group 51, Mississippi Department of Health.

80. Bessie Anne Swearegan, Torrance, to Lucy Massey, 3 August 1946, ibid.

81. The Board of Health employed the following black public health nurses: Eliza Farish Pillars, Beatrice Holmes, Gertrude Hughes, Florence Johnson, Gertrude Perkins, and Nettye Perkins. See 1936, box 36, Record Group 51, Mississippi Department of Health; and newsclipping from the *Jackson Clarion*, 4 April 1936, and scrapbooks, in the unprocessed Felix J. Underwood Papers, current Mississippi Department of Health, Jackson, Miss. I thank Theresa Hanna and Connie Bourgeois for making available the unprocessed papers of Underwood. See also Mary Elizabeth Carnegie, *The Path We Tread: Blacks in Nursing, 1854–1984* (Philadelphia: J. B. Lippincott, 1986), 35.

82. Midwife leader of club in Claiborne County, in Mississippi State Board of Health, "The Relation of the Midwife to the State Board of Health," 1 January 1935.

83. Leatha Johnson to Board of Health (1935?), box 27, Record Group 51, Mississippi Department of Health.

84. Celia Hall to Mary D. Osborne, 23 December 1936, box 27, and several photos of a Holmes County midwife meeting, October 1938, including photo of nurse Eliza Pillars with midwives, all in box 27, Record Group 51, Mississippi Department of Health.

85. Mississippi State Board of Health, "Midwife Supervision" (1938?), box 331, Central File, 1925–1928, Record Group 102, Children's Bureau; Felix Joel Underwood and Richard Noble Whitfield, *Public Health and Medical Licensure in the State of Mississippi, 1938–1947* (Jackson, Miss.: Tucker Printing House, 1951), 105; entry by Bess Blackwell on Eliza Farish Pillars for the "Biennial Nursing Hall of Fame Award of the Mississippi Nurses' Association," 1986 (courtesy of Edna Roberts), author's possession; George Alexander Sewell and Margaret L. Dwight, *Mississippi Black History Makers* (Jackson: University Press of Mississippi, 1977, rev. ed. 1984), 365–66; Carnegie, *The Path We Tread*, 159.

86. Nurse Permelia Harris, Yazoo County, "Mississippi State Board of Health,

Bureau of Child Hygiene and Public Health Nursing, Public Health Nurses' Narrative Reports," July 1928, box 41, Record Group 90, USPHS.

87. Nurse Ethel B. Marsh, Adams County, and itinerant nurse Eliza F. Pillars, in "Nurses Narrative Report, Mississippi State Board of Health, Bureau of Child Hygiene, Division of Public Health Nursing, July 1931," box 36, Record Group 51, Mississippi Department of Health.

88. Roberts, interview by the author.

89. Dodd, "Midwife Supervision in South Carolina," 863; "Educational Facilities For Colored Nurses and Their Employment," *Public Health Nursing* 17 (April 1925): 203; Nina D. Gage and Alma Haupt, "Some Observations on Negro Nursing in the South," *Public Health Nurse* 24 (December 1932): 676; Susie, *In the Way of Our Grandmothers*. See also Carter Godwin Woodson, *The Negro Professional Man and the Community* (Washington, D.C.: Association for the Study of Negro Life and History, 1934), 138, 140.

90. Grace Abbott to Salina Shaw, 9 December 1930, Central File, 1929–1932, box 367; Dr. Blanche Haines to Helen Bond, 20 June 1927, Central File, 1925–1928, box 279, both in Record Group 102, Children's Bureau. See also Dr. Montague Cobb, interview by the author, Washington D.C., 26 July 1989; Gloria Moldow, *Women Doctors in Gilded-Age Washington: Race, Gender, and Professionalization* (Urbana: University of Illinois, 1987), 26, 132; Rosalyn Terborg-Penn, "Ionia R. Whipper," in *Dictionary of American Negro Biography*, ed. Rayford W. Logan and Michael R. Winston (New York: W. W. Norton, 1982), 642–43.

91. Unknown midwife to Mary Osborne, 4 April 1938, box 27, Record Group 51, Mississippi Department of Health.

92. One must be careful not to overdraw the respect the Board of Health in general, and nurses in particular, held for midwives. For example, the nursing division of the health board had a habit of collecting lists of examples of midwife illiteracy, drawn from midwife club reports. Typewritten sheet of quotes, n.d., box 27, Record Group 51, Mississippi Department of Health.

93. Underwood, "Midwife Activities in Mississippi" [1932?], box 354; and Mississippi Department of Health, "Policies Regarding Midwife Supervision," 1 June 1948, box 36, Record Group 51, Mississippi Department of Health.

94. Molly Ladd-Taylor, "Women's Health and Public Policy," in *Women, Health, and Medicine in America*, ed. Apple, 398; Linda Gordon, *Heroes of Their Own Lives: The Politics and History of Family Violence* (New York: Viking, 1988), especially Introduction.

95. "Report of Work of Mollie Gilmore, Midwife, For July 1936 to December 1937," box 27, Record Group 51, Mississippi Department of Health.

96. Dr. W. E. Riecken, Jr., written responses to author; Ferguson, "Mississippi Midwives," 89.

97. Hall and Bourg, Sharkey-Issaquena Counties, "Nurses Narrative Report."

98. Midwife training film "All My Babies," Georgia Department of Health, 1953 (courtesy of the Department of the History of Medicine, University of Wisconsin Medical School).

99. Wilson, *Hope and Dignity*, 43. See also Schaffer, "The Health and Social Functions," 89–90, 98–99.

100. Midwife Estelle W. Christian to Nurse Viola M. Jones, Claiborne County, 5 October 1939, box 27, Record Group 51, Mississippi Department of Health.

101. Ibid. See also attached note from Jones to Osborne, box 27, Record Group 51, Mississippi Department of Health.

102. *Annual Report of the USPHS* (1925), 246. See also *Annual Report of the USPHS* (1922), 300; *Annual Report of the USPHS* (1926), 263; *Annual Report of the USPHS* (1927), 287.

103. Mississippi State Board of Health, "The Relation of the Midwife to the State Board of Health," 1 January 1944.

104. Letter from unknown midwife, Raleigh, to Board of Health, n.d., box 27; and Nurse Fannie Mae Howell, Holmes County, "Nurses Narrative Report, Mississippi State Board of Health, Bureau of Child Hygiene, Division of Public Health Nursing, July 1931," box 36, Record Group 51, Mississippi Department of Health.

105. Nurse Ethel B. Marsh, Adams County, "Nurses Narrative Report, Mississippi State Board of Health, Bureau of Child Hygiene, Division of Public Health Nursing, July 1931," box 36, Record Group 51, Mississippi Department of Health.

106. Nurse Nell E. Austin, Forrest County, ibid.

107. Nurse Edna U. Edwards, Pearl River County, "Nurses Narrative Report."

108. Connie Peak Higdon, Copiah County, "Nurses Narrative Report."

109. Folder, "Midwifery, Nursing Conference at Massey Island, Leflore County," September 1937, box 27, Record Group 51, Mississippi Department of Health.

110. Mississippi State Board of Health, "The Relation of the Midwife to the State Board of Health," 1 January 1935. See also nurse Mary L. Gregory, "Narrative and Statistical Report, April 1924, Mississippi State Board of Health, Bureau of Child Hygiene and Public Health Nursing," Central File, 1921–1924, box 249, Record Group 102, Children's Bureau.

111. Midwife leader in Smith County, quoted in Mississippi State Board of Health, "The Relation of the Midwife to the State Board of Health," 1 January 1935.

112. Nurse Ella M. Sayle, Coahoma County, Mississippi State Board of Health, Bureau of Child Hygiene and Public Health Nursing, Public Health Nurses' Narrative Reports, July 1928, box 41, Record Group 90, USPHS.

113. Nurses' reports in "The Relation of the Midwife to the State Board of Health," 1 January 1935.

114. Midwife Virginia Thompson, Hamilton, Monroe County to Mary D. Osborne, 21 July 1936, box 27, Record Group 51, Mississippi Department of Health.

115. Underwood, "Midwife Activities in Mississippi" [1932?], box 354, Record Group 51, Mississippi Department of Health; "The Relation of the Midwife to the State Board of Health," 1 January 1935.

116. Litoff, *American Midwives*, 51.

117. Midwife report from Simpson County, n.d. [1930s or 1940s], box 27, Record Group 51, Mississippi Department of Health.

118. Letter from unknown midwife to Board of Health, n.d., box 36, Record Group 51, Mississippi Department of Health.

119. Photo of a midwife and Mrs. Robley, possibly the nurse, showing a

delivery room, n.d., box 21; photo entitled "Model Midwife Delivery Room" in Sharkey County, 1953, box 36; sketch of a model delivery room, n.d., box 27; Nurse Elois Conn, *Southern Herald*, 12 November [1941?], box 27, all in Record Group 51, Mississippi Department of Health. Note the similarities to the Kelly pad described by Judith Leavitt in *Brought to Bed*, 273, and illustration, 62.

120. Mississippi State Board of Health, "The Relation of the Midwife to the State Board of Health," 1 January 1935; newsclipping "Midwives and Health Work" [1933?], box 36; Mississippi State Board of Health, "Midwife Supervision" [1938?], box 36, all in Record Group 51, Mississippi Department of Health. See also Roberts, interview by the author.

121. J. M. Boyd to Mary D. Osborne, 24 May 1934, box 27, Record Group 51, Mississippi Department of Health.

122. Excerpts from testimony about model delivery rooms, box 27, Record Group 51, Mississippi Department of Health.

123. Mrs. B. S. Peques, Itta Bena, to Board of Health, n.d., box 27, Record Group 51, Mississippi Department of Health.

124. Dr. B. B. Harper, Itta Bena, to Mary Osborne, 6 May 1938, box 27, Record Group 51, Mississippi Department of Health.

125. Comments by Mrs. Elliott Thompson and Mat Jones about delivery room set up by Lula B. Hudson at Rust College, 6 August 1941, box 27, Record Group 51, Mississippi Department of Health.

126. Brooksie W. Peters, for the nursing staff of the Lauderdale County Health Department, to Lucy E. Massey, 14 July 1947, box 36; and Dr. Andrew Hedmeg, Jackson County Health Department, reporting on nurses' suggestions to Lucy E. Massey, 8 September 1947, box 36, Record Group 51, Mississippi Department of Health. Florida's midwife retirement efforts also began in the 1940s. Susie, *In the Way of Our Grandmothers*, 51.

127. Mississippi State Board of Health, "Policies Regarding Midwife Supervision," 1 June 1948, box 36; memo from Lucy Massey to Dr. Underwood, 2 February 1948, and memo from Underwood to Massey, 2 February 1948, box 36, Record Group 51, Mississippi Department of Health.

128. Roberts, interview by the author.

129. Loftus, "Stork Loses Two Long-Time Forrest County Helpers."

130. Dr. D. Galloway and Nurse Louise Holmes, Mississippi State Board of Health, to Dr. Lucille Marsh, Children's Bureau, 3 December 1951, box 36, Record Group 51, Mississippi Department of Health.

131. Roberts, interview by the author.

132. In 1951 there were only about 30 white midwives. Dr. D. Galloway and Nurse Louise Holmes, Mississippi State Board of Health, to Dr. Lucille Marsh, Children's Bureau, 3 December 1951; "State Health Agency Calls Midwifery 'Dying Avocation'"; note to Miss Ferguson on midwife figures as of December 1975, all in box 36, Record Group 51, Mississippi Department of Health. See also "Grannies: The roots of midwifery"; Jelks, "My Twenty-Five Years in Public Health"; and Roberts, interview by the author. A similar pattern held in Florida, with only a few registered midwives by the 1980s. Susie, *In the Way of Our Grandmothers*, 55; and for Texas, see Schaffer, "The Health and Social Functions," 100.

Chapter 6

1. In the 1950s, southern historian C. Vann Woodward referred to the "New Reconstruction" that begin in the 1930s and reached full momentum after World War II. C. Vann Woodward, *The Strange Career of Jim Crow* (New York: Oxford University Press, 1957), 9. There is much debate among historians over the extent to which New Deal measures benefited African Americans. See Raymond Wolters, *Negroes and the Great Depression: The Problem of Economic Recovery* (Westport, Conn.: Greenwood Press, 1970); Harvard Sitkoff, *A New Deal for Blacks: The Emergence of Civil Rights as a National Issue* (New York: Oxford University Press, 1978), especially chapter 2; Edward H. Beardsley, *A History of Neglect: Health Care for Blacks and Mill Workers in the Twentieth-Century South* (Knoxville: University of Tennessee Press, 1987), chapter 7.

2. Background information on the Alpha Kappa Alpha Sorority and the Mississippi Health Project was drawn from Marjorie H. Parker, *Alpha Kappa Alpha: 60 Years of Service* (n.p.: Alpha Kappa Alpha Sorority, 1966); J. D. Ratcliff, "Cotton Field Clinic," *Survey Graphic* 29 (September 1940): 464–67. For a history of another black sorority see Paula Giddings, *In Search of Sisterhood: Delta Sigma Theta and the Challenge of the Black Sorority Movement* (New York: William Morrow, 1988).

3. Ratcliff, "Cotton Field Clinic," 464–67; *Alpha Kappa Alpha Mississippi Health Project, Annual Report* [hereinafter *AKAMHP, Annual Report*] (1935), available at Howard University, Moorland-Spingarn Research Center, Washington, D.C.; *AKAMHP, Annual Report* (1938); and *AKAMHP, Annual Report* (1939); Sitkoff, *A New Deal for Blacks*, 98; Pete Daniel, *Standing at the Crossroads: Southern Life Since 1900* (New York: Hill and Wang, 1986), 84.

4. Ida Louise Jackson, quoted in James Willis Jackson [no relation], "The Search for Something Better: Ida Louise Jackson's Life Story," 204, unpublished manuscript (courtesy of James W. Jackson).

5. *AKAMHP, Annual Report* (1935), Foreword. See also J. Jackson, "Search for Something Better," 174–75.

6. *AKAMHP, Annual Report* (1935), Foreword.

7. *AKAMHP, Annual Report* (1937), Foreword.

8. "Concerning the Health Project," *Ivy Leaf* 16 (December 1938): 49. See also Gerda Lerner, "Community Work of Black Club Women," *The Majority Finds Its Past: Placing Women in History* (New York: Oxford University Press, 1979), 93; Deborah Gray White, "The Cost of Club Work, the Price of Black Feminism," in *Visible Women: New Essays on American Activism*, ed. Nancy A. Hewitt and Suzanne Lebsock (Urbana: University of Illinois Press, 1993), 260.

9. Jackson quoted in J. Jackson, "Search for Something Better," 30, and see 253. See also "Ida Louise Jackson," *Ivy Leaf* 57 (Spring 1980): 10; Marianna Davis, ed., *Contributions of Black Women to America*, vol. 2 (Columbia, S.C.: Kenday Press, 1982), 406; "Ida L. Jackson," in *There Was Light: Autobiography of a University, Berkeley: 1868–1968* ed. Irving Stone (New York: Doubleday, 1970), 249–66.

10. Arenia C. Mallory King headed the school, later called Saints Junior College, from 1926 to 1983. "Ida Louise Jackson"; Davis, *Contributions of Black Women*,

406; Stone, "Ida L. Jackson"; J. Jackson, "Search for Something Better," 166–68, 174.

11. J. Jackson, "Search for Something Better," 202.

12. Ratcliff, "Cotton Field Clinic," 465; Ida L. Jackson, "My Reflections on Alpha Kappa Alpha's Summer School For Rural Teachers and the Mississippi Health Project," *Ivy Leaf* 52 (Summer 1976): 11; Parker, *Alpha Kappa Alpha*, 101–2; "Lexington: A Noble Task," *Ivy Leaf* 13 (March 1935): 12; and J. Jackson, "Search for Something Better," 175–79, 181, 201–2.

13. J. Jackson, "Search for Something Better," 183.

14. *AKAMHP, Annual Report* (1935); J. Jackson, "Search for Something Better," 177, 180, 182, 188.

15. Carolyn Lewis, interview with Dr. Ferebee, "Hard Work Can Topple the Barriers," *Washington Post*, n.d. (located in folder on Dr. Dorothy Ferebee, Howardiana Collection, Howard University Archives, Moorland-Spingarn Research Center, Howard University, Washington, D.C.).

16. Biographical information on Ferebee drawn from Davis, *Contributions of Black Women*, 407; "A Thumbnail Sketch of Our Supreme Basileus Dorothy Boulding Ferebee," *Ivy Leaf* 18 (March 1940): 4; "Dorothy Boulding Ferebee," *Tufts Medical Alumni Bulletin* 27 (March 1968) (located in folder on Dr. Dorothy Ferebee, Health Sciences Library, Howard University).

17. Dorothy Boulding Ferebee to Ida Louise Jackson, 30 June 1935, box 10, Dorothy Ferebee Papers, Manuscript Division, Moorland-Spingarn Research Center, Howard University; K. E. Miller to Dr. J. A. O'Hara, 19 March 1937, general records 1936–1944, box 147, Record Group 90, United States Public Health Service (USPHS); "Negro College Women Conduct Health Project in Delta," *National Negro Health News* 8 (October–December 1940): 26.

18. Biographical information on Williams in "An Appreciation," *Ivy Leaf* 15 (March 1937): 19; "Soror Mary Williams, *Ivy Leaf* 16 (September 1938): 7–8; *Southern Letter* 43 (August 1927): 2–3.

19. Mary Williams to Dorothy Boulding Ferebee, 18 March 1935, box 10, Ferebee Papers.

20. Dr. Dorothy Ferebee, "The Alpha Kappa Alpha Mississippi Health Project," *Ivy Leaf* 52 (Summer 1976): 14.

21. Jackson quoted in J. Jackson, "Search for Something Better," 190.

22. Dorothy Boulding Ferebee, interview by Merze Tate, 28 and 31 December 1979, Arthur and Elizabeth Schlesinger Library in the History of Women in America, Radcliffe College, in vol. 3, Ruth Edmonds Hill, ed., *The Black Women Oral History Project* (Westport, Conn.: Meckler, 1991), 466, 433–81. See also *AKAMHP, Annual Report* (1935); Jackson, "My Reflections," 11–13.

23. The Holmes County health officer had warned Ferebee that transportation difficulties meant it was "entirely impractical" to expect mothers and children to come to one clinic location. C. J. Vaughn to Dorothy Boulding Ferebee, 25 June 1935; and Dorothy Boulding Ferebee to Arenia Mallory, 22 June 1935, box 10, Ferebee Papers.

24. Ida Louise Jackson to Dorothy Boulding Ferebee, 17 June 1935; Mary

Williams to Dorothy Boulding Ferebee, 3 November 1935; Marion Carter to Dorothy Ferebee, 18 December 1935; Dorothy Boulding Ferebee to Florence Alexander, 27 June 1936; Marion Carter to Dorothy Boulding Ferebee, 18 July 1936, all in box 10, Ferebee Papers.

25. Ella Payne Moran, "A Project conducted in Mississippi, Alpha Kappa Alpha Sorority Health Project, Mississippi, 1935–1942," paper for an education course at Howard University, August 1942, p. 3; "Impressions of Mound Bayou by Staff Nurse," 1936; Rosier Dedwylder to Dorothy Boulding Ferebee, 14 April 1936, all in box 10, Ferebee Papers; "Lexington: A Noble Task"; Dr. Martha Eliot to Dr. Felix Underwood, 19 February 1937, box 133, Correspondence and Reports Relating to Surveys, 1917–1954, Record Group 102, Children's Bureau, National Archives, Washington, D.C.

26. *AKAMHP, Annual Report* (1941), box 10, Ferebee Papers; Ida Louise Jackson, interview by the author, 27 September 1990, telephone; Ratcliff, "Cotton Field Clinic," 464–67; J. Jackson, "Search for Something Better," 192–93.

27. Ferebee, interview, *The Black Women Oral History Project*, 466.

28. Ida Louise Jackson, "A Message from Our Supreme Basileus," *Ivy Leaf* 13 (September 1935): 3–4.

29. I. Jackson, "My Reflections," 13.

30. J. Jackson, "Search for Something Better," 191, 232.

31. Parker, *Alpha Kappa Alpha*, 106. See also, I. Jackson, "A Message."

32. Ida Jackson to Dorothy Ferebee, n.d. [early 1935?], box 10, Ferebee Papers.

33. Mary E. Williams to Dr. Paraham, 31 July 1937; A. J. Aselmeyer to Mary E. Williams, 10 August 1937, Group 9, general records, box 64, Record Group 90, USPHS; Dorothy Ferebee to Dr. Raymond Vonderlehr, 4 August 1938, Group 3, States 1936–1944, Mississippi, Record Group 90, USPHS. See also J. Jackson, "Search for Something Better," 210, 230.

34. *AKAMHP, Annual Report* (1936); typescript by Marjorie Holloman, 1936, box 10, Ferebee Papers.

35. Helen Kitchen Branson, *Let There Be Light: The Contemporary Account of Edna L. Griffin, M.D.* (Pasadena, Calif.: M. S. Sen, 1947), 103.

36. Mississippi State Board of Health, "The Relation of the Midwife to the State Board of Health," 1 January 1935, box 2, Record Group 51, Mississippi Department of Health, Mississippi Department of Archives and History, Jackson, Miss.; Ratcliff, "Cotton Field Clinic."

37. "Deplorable Health Conditions Down in Mississippi Revealed by Doctor Who Conducted AKA Project," newsclipping from unknown Washington, D.C., newspaper, 22 November 1935, box 10, Ferebee Papers.

38. My thanks to Vanessa Northington Gamble for helping to clarify my thinking on this point.

39. Report by unknown sorority member, 1936, box 10, Ferebee Papers.

40. Moran, "A Project conducted in Mississippi," 3.

41. Dr. Dorothy Ferebee, "Proposed Plan for a Demonstrational Dietotherapy Project by the Alpha Kappa Alpha Sorority Health Unit," p. 6, box 10, Ferebee Papers; *AKAMHP, Annual Report* (1939).

42. Ferebee, "The Alpha Kappa Alpha Mississippi Health Project," 15.

43. Ruth A. Scott, "Life's Blood in Mississippi," *Ivy Leaf* 18 (September 1940): 5.

44. Parker, *Alpha Kappa Alpha*, 104–7. See also *AKAMHP, Annual Report* (1935–1942).

45. Ratcliff, "Cotton Field Clinic," 467; "Mound Bayou Erects New Model in Community Health," *Philadelphia Afro-American*, 3 March 1946, p. 5; I. Jackson, interview by the author; Florence Warfield Sillers, *History of Bolivar County, Mississippi* (Jackson, Miss.: Hederman Brothers, 1948), 249; Herbert M. Morais, *The History of the Negro in Medicine* (New York: Publishers Company for the Association for the Study of Negro Life and History, 1967), 149.

46. Moran, "A Project in Mississippi," 5–12.

47. Griffin, in Branson, *Let There Be Light*, 105.

48. *AKAMHP, Annual Report* (1942), 21, see also 18.

49. *AKAMHP, Annual Report* (1935), Appendix.

50. *AKAMHP, Annual Report* (1937), 16–17.

51. Scott, "Life's Blood in Mississippi," 5.

52. See critiques of sharecropping in the *AKAMHP, Annual Report* (1937).

53. *AKAMHP, Annual Report* (1941), Foreword.

54. *AKAMHP, Annual Report* (1941).

55. See Parker, *Alpha Kappa Alpha*, 111–12; Ferebee, "The Alpha Kappa Alpha Mississippi Health Project," 15; and Flora B. Chisholm, "Full-time Health Education Program of the Alpha Kappa Alpha Sorority," *National Negro Health News* 15 (October-December 1947): 11–13; I. Jackson, interview by the author. Biographical information on Estelle Massey Riddle Osborne in Darlene Clark Hine, *Black Women in White: Racial Conflict and Cooperation in the Nursing Profession, 1890–1950* (Bloomington: Indiana University Press, 1989), 97, 118–19.

56. Roscoe C. Brown to Dorothy Boulding Ferebee, 27 February 1935, box 10, Ferebee Papers.

57. Some of this correspondence is reproduced in *AKAMHP, Annual Report* (1935). See also AKA folder in Group 9, general records 1936–1944, Organizations, box 147, Record Group 90, USPHS; Mississippi folder, Correspondence and Reports 1917–1952, box 133, Record Group 102, Children's Bureau.

58. "Ida Louise Jackson," 10; Jackson, "My Reflections," 13; *Ivy Leaf* 14 (March 1936): 23; Stone, "Ida L. Jackson," 201.

59. Ida L. Jackson, "The Conference with Mrs. Roosevelt," *Ivy Leaf* 14 (June 1936): 4.

60. I. Jackson, "The Conference with Mrs. Roosevelt," 4.

61. *AKAMHP Annual Report* (1937), 9. See also *AKAMHP, Annual Report* (1938), Foreword; J. Jackson, "Search for Something Better," 225.

62. I. Jackson quoted in J. Jackson, "Search for Something Better," 231.

63. Ida Louise Jackson to Dr. Martha Eliot, 17 May 1943; Dr. Van Riper to Dr. Martha Eliot, 24 May 1943; Dr. Beach to Dr. Van Riper, 19 July 1943, Central File 1941–1944, box 35, Record Group 102, Children's Bureau. See also William I. Trattner, *From Poor Law to Welfare State: A History of Social Welfare in America* (New York: The Free Press, 1989), 199–200.

64. Photo album with text by Portia Nickens, box 10, Ferebee Papers; Dorothy Ferebee, "A Message From Our Supreme Basileus," *Ivy Leaf* 18 (December 1940): 3; quote from Frederick Douglass in "The Alpha Kappa Alpha Sorority Continues Health Project and Establishes National Non-Partisan Council," *Aframerican Woman's Journal* 1 (1941): 38.

65. The other organizations were Alpha Phi Alpha, Delta Sigma Theta, Phi Beta Sigma, Sigma Gamma Rho, and Zeta Phi Beta. "American Council on Human Rights," folder 1274, box 57, National Association for the Advancement of Colored People, Washington D.C., Branch Collection, Manuscript Division, Moorland-Spingarn Research Center.

66. Bettye Collier-Thomas, *N.C.N.W., 1935–1980* (Washington, D.C.: National Council of Negro Women, 1981), 1–4. See also the journal of the National Council of Negro Women, *Aframerican Woman's Journal*.

67. Mary McLeod Bethune, "My Secret Talks with FDR," *Ebony* 6 (April 1949): 43–51; Collier-Thomas, *N.C.N.W.*, 1–4; Rackham Holt, *Mary McLeod Bethune: A Biography* (Garden City, N.Y.: Doubleday, 1964); B. Joyce Ross, "Mary McLeod Bethune and the National Youth Administration: A Case Study of Power Relationships in the Black Cabinet of Franklin D. Roosevelt," in *Black Leaders of the Twentieth Century* ed. John Hope Franklin and August Meier (Urbana: University of Illinois Press, 1982), 191–219.

68. On Council health activities, see Records of the National Council of Negro Women, Series 5, boxes 15 and 16, Subject Files, 1942–1949, Bethune Museum and Archives, Washington, D.C.; and *Aframerican Woman's Journal* 1 (Spring 1940): back cover.

69. Susan Ware, *Beyond Suffrage: Women in the New Deal* (Cambridge, Mass.: Harvard University Press, 1981), 12.

70. Information on Vinita Lewis contained in Central File 1941–1944, box 35, Record Group 102, Children's Bureau.

71. Hallie Q. Brown and two other women on the Republican National Committee, after helping to elect President Calvin Coolidge in 1924, wrote Coolidge requesting that black women receive positions in the federal government currently only held by white women, including in the Department of Labor, the Children's Bureau, the Bureau of Education, and the Department of Agriculture. Hallie Q. Brown, M. C. Lawton, and Myrtle Foster to President Calvin Coolidge, 6 May 1925, Correspondence 1924–1939, Negroes, box 2, Record Group 16, Office of the Secretary of Agriculture, National Archives.

72. Proceedings of the "White House Conference of the National Council of Negro Women, Inc., Monday, April 4, 1938," Records of the National Council of Negro Women, Series 4, box 1.

73. See photo of the women in *Aframerican Woman's Journal* 1 (Spring 1940): 5.

74. The government administrators who attended were Lawrence A. Oxley of the Department of Labor, Robert C. Weaver and Frank S. Horne of the U.S. Housing Authority, Ellen S. Woodward of the Works Progress Administration, Dr. Louise Stanley of the Bureau of Home Economics in the Department of Agriculture, Mary Anderson of the Women's Bureau, Katharine Lenroot of the Children's

Bureau, Atha C. Jordan of the National Youth Administration, and Mary (Molly) Dewson of the Social Security Board. "The National Council of Negro Women of The United States of America, Inc.," *Aframerican Woman's Journal* 1 (Spring 1940): 3; "Large Group of Alpha Kappa Alpha Women Attend" and "Conference on the Participation of Negro Women and Children in Federal Welfare Programs," *Ivy Leaf* 16 (June 1938): 3–4; and form letter from Bethune, 17 March 1938, and agenda, both in Records of the National Council of Negro Women, Series 4, box 1.

75. Proceedings, p. 6.

76. Sitkoff, *A New Deal for Blacks*, 52.

77. Proceedings, p. 89.

78. Bethune, Proceedings, p. 13 (emphasis in original).

79. Dorothy Boulding Ferebee to Zenobia Gilpin, 27 June 1935, box 10, Ferebee Papers.

80. Ella V. Payne to Dorothy Ferebee, 9 October 1935, box 10, Ferebee Papers.

81. Photo album, box 10, Ferebee Papers; "Supreme Basileus Recipient of Award," *Ivy Leaf* 18 (December 1940): 4; Parker, *Alpha Kappa Alpha*, 105.

82. For an example of Ferebee's publicity work, see *Philadelphia Afro-American*, 30 March 1940, p. 9.

83. Bessie E. Cobbs, "Health on Wheels in Mississippi," *American Journal of Nursing* 41 (May 1941): 551–54.

84. Zatella R. Turner, "Alpha Kappa Alpha Sorority's Wartime Program," *The Aframerican Woman's Journal* 3 (Summer 1943): 22.

85. Lawrence J. Nelson, "Welfare Capitalism on a Mississippi Plantation in the Great Depression," *Journal of Southern History* 50 (May 1984): 225.

86. Ida Jackson to Dorothy Ferebee, 2 June 1936, box 10, Ferebee Papers.

87. Ferebee, "The Alpha Kappa Alpha Mississippi Health Project," 15.

88. Dr. Dorothy Ferebee, "A Brief Review of the Mississippi Health Project of the Alpha Kappa Alpha Sorority," presented 10 February 1973, at the 65th anniversary of AKA, box 12, Ferebee Papers.

Conclusion

1. Harvard Sitkoff, "The Impact of the New Deal on Black Southerners," in *The New Deal and the South: Essays*, ed. James C. Cobb and Michael V. Namorato (Jackson: University Press of Mississippi, 1984), 117–34. See also James C. Cobb, "'Somebody Done Nailed Us on the Cross': Federal Farm and Welfare Policy and the Civil Rights Movement in the Mississippi Delta," *Journal of American History* 77 (December 1990): 912–36.

2. My thanks to Nellie McKay for her insights on this point.

3. Marie A. Laberge, "'We Are Proud of Our Gains': Wisconsin Black Women's Organizational Work in the Post World War II Period," paper presented at the Berkshire Conference on Women's History, June 1990, Rutgers University, New Brunswick, N.J., author's possession.

4. Herbert M. Morais, *The History of the Negro in Medicine* (New York: Publishers Company for the Association for the Study of Negro Life and History,

1967), chapters 8–10; Darlene Clark Hine, *Black Women in White: Racial Conflict and Cooperation in the Nursing Profession, 1890–1950* (Bloomington: Indiana University Press, 1989), 184, 192.

5. Nancy Krieger, "Shades of Difference: Theoretical Underpinnings of the Medical Controversy on Black/White Differences in the United States, 1830–1870," *International Journal of Health Services* 17, no. 2 (1987): 275–76; Angela Davis, "Sick and Tired of Being Sick and Tired: The Politics of Black Women's Health," in *The Black Women's Health Book: Speaking for Ourselves*, ed. Evelyn C. White (Seattle: Seal Press, 1990), 19–26.

6. Davis, "Sick and Tired," 20; Andrea Lewis, "Looking at the Total Picture: A Conversation with Health Activist Beverly Smith," in *The Black Women's Health Book*, 174–77. See also bell hooks, *Sisters of the Yam: Black Women and Self-Recovery* (Boston: South End Press, 1993).

7. Linda Asantewaa Johnson, "Black Women's Health Issues," *Off Our Backs* 13, no. 8 (August/September 1983): 12–13; Betty Norwood Chaney, "Black Women's Health Conference," *Southern Changes* 5, no. 5 (October/November 1983): 18–20.

8. The Smithsonian lecture series was a product of Vital Signs in association with the African American Studies Program of the Smithsonian Institution and the Urban Health Program of the University of Illinois.

Selected Bibliography

MANUSCRIPT COLLECTIONS

Howard University, Moorland-Spingarn Research Center, Washington, D.C.
    Dorothy Ferebee Papers
    Howardiana Collection
    Peter Marshall Murray Papers
    National Association for the Advancement of Colored People, Washington, D.C., Branch Collection
    Mabel Keaton Staupers Papers
    Mary Church Terrell Papers
    Louis T. Wright Papers
Library of Congress, Manuscript Division, Washington, D.C.
    Booker T. Washington Papers
    National Urban League Records
    National Urban League Southern Regional Division Records
Mississippi Department of Archives and History, Jackson.
    Department of Health, Record Group 51
    Subject Files
    Works Projects Administration, Record Group 60
Mississippi State Department of Health, Jackson
    Felix Underwood Papers
National Archives, Washington, D.C.
    Children's Bureau, Record Group 102
    Department of Health, Education and Welfare, Record Group 235
    Extension Service, Record Group 33
    Extension Service, Statistical and Narrative Reports, Alabama (1909–1917, 1920, 1923, 1930, 1935), Mississippi (1935–1942)
    Public Health Service, Record Group 90
    Office of the Secretary of Agriculture, Record Group 16
Bethune Museum and Archives, Washington, D.C.
    Records of the National Council of Negro Women
    Vertical Files
Washington Collection, Hollis Burke Frissell Library, Tuskegee University, Tuskegee, Alabama
    Thomas Monroe Campbell Papers
    Department of Records and Research Files
    Jessie P. Guzman Papers
    Albon L. Holsey Papers

Robert Russa Moton Papers
Tuskegee Institute Extension Service Collection
Tuskegee Institute News Clippings File
Margaret Murray Washington Papers
Monroe Nathan Work Papers

ORAL HISTORIES

Ruth Edmonds Hill, ed., *The Black Women Oral History Project*. Westport, Conn.:
    Meckler, 1991. From the Arthur and Elizabeth Schlesinger Library on the
    History of Women in America.
    Ferebee, Dorothy Boulding. Interview by Merze Tate, December 28 and 31,
        1979. Volume 3, pages 433–81.
    Laurie, Eunice Rivers. Interview by A. Lillian Thompson, October 10, 1977.
        Volume 7, pages 213–42.

INTERVIEWS

Brown Jr., Dr. Roscoe C. Telephone interview by author, 29 November 1988, New
    York. Interview notes.
Cobb, Dr. W. Montague. Interview by author, 26 July 1989, Washington, D.C.
    Interview notes.
Cornely, Dr. Paul. Interview by author, 24 July 1989, Howard University Medical
    School, Washington, D.C. Tape recording.
Guzman, Jessie. Interview by author, 10 September 1989, Tuskegee, Alabama. Tape
    recording.
Jackson, Ida Louise. Telephone interview by author, 27 September 1990, California.
    Interview notes.
Roberts, Edna. Interview by author, 17 September 1989, Jackson, Mississippi. Tape
    recording.
Staupers, Mabel Keaton. Interview by author, 30 July 1989, Washington, D.C.
    Interview notes.

ANNUAL REPORTS, NEWSPAPERS, AND PERIODICALS

Aframerican Woman's Journal (1940–1949)
Agricultural History (1927–1987)
Alpha Kappa Alpha Mississippi Health Project, Annual Report (1935–1942)
American Journal of Public Health (1915–1968)
Annual Report of Provident Hospital and Training School (1892–1915)
Annual Report of the Mississippi Board of Health (1909–1951)
Annual Report of the Surgeon General of the Public Health Service of the United States
    (1917–1955)

Crisis (1911–1980)
Ebony (1945–1980)
Howard Medical News [later the *National Medical News*] (1924–1941)
Ivy Leaf (1921–1950, 1976, 1980)
Journal of Negro Education (1932–1986)
Journal of Southern History (1936–1990)
Journal of the National Medical Association (1909–1955)
National Negro Health News (1933–1950)
National Notes (1904, 1908, 1911–1924, 1927–1930, 1933, 1947–1948, 1953)
Philadelphia Afro-American (1935–1950)
Phylon (1960–1986)
Proceedings of the National Negro Business League (1915–1919, 1921, 1924, 1940)
Public Health Nurse (1924–1941)
Rural Messenger (1920–1924)
Southern Letter (1915–1931)
Southern Workman (1910–1939)
Tuskegeean (1930–1931, 1939–1941)

BOOKS

Anderson, James D. *The Education of Blacks in the South, 1860–1935*. Chapel Hill: University of North Carolina Press, 1988.

Apple, Rima D., ed. *Women, Health and Medicine in America: A Historical Handbook*. New York: Garland, 1990.

Baker, Gladys L. *The County Agent*. Chicago: University of Chicago Press, 1939.

Beard, Mary Ritter. *Woman's Work in Municipalities*. New York: D. Appleton, 1915.

Beardsley, Edward H. *A History of Neglect: Health Care for Blacks and Mill Workers in the Twentieth-Century South*. Knoxville: University of Tennessee Press, 1987.

Brandt, Allan M. *No Magic Bullet: A Social History of Venereal Disease in the United States Since 1880*. New York: Oxford University Press, 1987.

Branson, Helen Kitchen. *Let There Be Light: The Contemporary Account of Edna L. Griffin, M.D.* Pasadena, Calif.: M. S. Sen, 1947.

Brown, E. Richard. *Rockefeller Medicine Men: Medicine and Capitalism in America*. Berkeley: University of California Press, 1979.

Buckler, Helen. *Daniel Hale Williams, Negro Surgeon*. New York: Pitman, 1954. Reprint 1968.

Buhler-Wilkerson, Karen. *False Dawn: The Rise and Decline of Public Health Nursing, 1900–1930*. New York: Garland, 1989.

——, ed. *Nursing and the Public's Health: An Anthology of Sources*. New York: Garland, 1989.

Campbell, Marie. *Folks Do Get Born*. New York: Rinehart, 1946.

Campbell, Thomas Monroe. *The Movable School Goes to the Negro Farmer*. Tuskegee, Ala.: Tuskegee Institute Press, 1936. Reprint New York: Arno Press and the New York Times, 1969.

Carnegie, Mary Elizabeth. *The Path We Tread: Blacks in Nursing, 1854–1984*. Philadelphia: J. B. Lippincott, 1986.

Cobb, James C. and Michael V. Namorato, eds. *The New Deal and the South: Essays*. Jackson: University Press of Mississippi, 1984.

Collier-Thomas, Bettye. *N.C.N.W., 1935–1980*. Washington, D.C.: National Council of Negro Women, 1981.

Daniel, Pete. *The Shadow of Slavery: Peonage in the South, 1901–1969*. Urbana: University of Illinois Press, 1972, 1990.

——. *Standing at the Crossroads: Southern Life Since 1900*. New York: Hill and Wang, 1986.

Dannett, Sylvia G.L., *Profiles of Negro Womanhood*. 2 vols. Yonkers, N.Y.: Negro Heritage Library, Educational Heritage, 1966.

Davis, Elizabeth Lindsay. *Lifting as They Climb*. Washington, D.C.: National Association of Colored Women, 1933.

Davis, Marianna W., ed. *Contributions of Black Women to America*. 2 vols. Columbia, S.C.: Kenday Press, 1982.

Du Bois, W.E.B. *The Autobiography of W.E.B. Du Bois*. New York: International Publishers, 1968.

——, ed. *Efforts for Social Betterment Among Negro Americans*. Atlanta University Publication no. 3. Atlanta: Atlanta University Press, 1898.

——, ed. *Efforts for Social Betterment Among Negro Americans*. Atlanta University Publication no. 14. Atlanta: Atlanta University Press, 1909.

——, ed. *The Health Physique of the Negro American*. Atlanta University Publication no. 11. Atlanta: Atlanta University Press, 1906.

Dummett, Clifton O. and Lois Doyle. *Afro-Americans in Dentistry: Sequence and Consequence of Events*. n.p.: Clifton Dummett, 1978.

Ellis, John H. *Yellow Fever and Public Health in the New South*. Lexington: University Press of Kentucky, 1992.

Etheridge, Elizabeth W. *The Butterfly Caste: A Social History of Pellagra in the South*. Westport, Conn.: Greenwood Press, 1972.

Ettling, John. *The Germ of Laziness: Rockefeller Philanthropy and Public Health in the New South*. Cambridge, Mass.: Harvard University Press, 1981.

Fleming, G. James and Christian E. Burckel, ed. *Who's Who in Colored America*. 7th edition. Yonkers-on-Hudson, New York: Christian E. Burckel & Associates, 1950.

Flexner, Eleanor. *Century of Struggle: The Woman's Rights Movement in the United States*. Cambridge, Mass.: Belknap Press of Harvard University Press, 1959; rev. ed. 1975.

Furman, Bess. *A Profile of the United States Public Health Service, 1798–1948*. Washington, D.C.: U.S. Government Printing Office, 1973.

Gamble, Vanessa Northington. *The Black Community Hospital: Contemporary Dilemmas in Historical Perspective*. New York: Garland, 1989.

——, ed. *Germs Have No Color Line: Blacks and American Medicine, 1900–1940*. New York: Garland, 1989.

Gaus, John M. and Leon O. Wolcott. *Public Administration and the United States Department of Agriculture*. Chicago: 1940. Reprint New York: Da Capo Press, 1975.

Giddings, Paula. *In Search of Sisterhood: Delta Sigma Theta and the Challenge of the Black Sorority Movement*. New York: William Morrow, 1988.

———. *When and Where I Enter: The Impact of Black Women on Race and Sex in America*. New York: William Morrow, 1984.

Gordon, Linda. *Heroes of Their Own Lives: The Politics and History of Family Violence*. New York: Viking, 1988.

———, ed. *Women, the State, and Welfare*. Madison: University of Wisconsin Press, 1990.

Guzman, Jessie Parkhurst, ed. *The Negro Year Book, 1952: A Review of Events Affecting Negro Life*. New York: William H. Wise, 1952.

Harlan, Louis. *Booker T. Washington: The Making of a Black Leader, 1856–1901*. New York: Oxford University Press, 1972, 1983.

———. *Booker T. Washington: The Wizard of Tuskegee, 1901–1915*. New York: Oxford University Press, 1983.

Harley, Sharon and Rosalyn Terborg-Penn, eds. *The Afro-American Woman: Struggles and Images*. Port Washington, N.Y.: University Publications, Kennikat Press, 1978.

Haws, Robert, ed. *The Age of Segregation: Race Relations in the South, 1890–1945*. Jackson: University Press of Mississippi, 1978.

Hewitt, Nancy A. and Suzanne Lebsock, eds. *Visible Women: New Essays on American Activism*. Urbana: University of Illinois Press, 1993.

Higginbotham, Evelyn Brooks. *Righteous Discontent: The Women's Movement in the Black Baptist Church, 1880–1920*. Cambridge, Mass.: Harvard University Press, 1993.

Hine, Darlene Clark, ed. *Black Women in the Nursing Profession: A Documentary History*. New York: Garland, 1985.

———. *Black Women in White: Racial Conflict and Cooperation in the Nursing Profession, 1890–1950*. Bloomington: Indiana University Press, 1989.

———. *When the Truth Is Told: A History of Black Women's Culture and Community in Indiana, 1875–1950*. n.p.: National Council of Negro Women, 1981.

———, ed. *The State of Afro-American History: Past, Present, and Future*. Baton Rouge: Louisiana State University Press, 1986.

Hoffman, Frederick L. *Race Traits and Tendencies of the American Negro*. New York: Published for the American Economics Association by Macmillan, 1896.

Humphreys, Margaret. *Yellow Fever and the South*. New Brunswick, N.J.: Rutgers University Press, 1992.

Johnson, Charles S. *Shadow of the Plantation*. Chicago: University of Chicago Press, 1934.

Jones, Jacqueline. *Labor of Love, Labor of Sorrow: Black Women, Work, and the Family from Slavery to the Present*. New York: Basic Books, 1985.

Jones, James H. *Bad Blood: The Tuskegee Syphilis Experiment*. New York: Free Press, 1981. Expanded edition 1993.

Kenney, John A. *The Negro in Medicine*. By the author, 1912.

Ladd-Taylor, Molly. *Mother-Work: Women, Child Welfare, and the State, 1890–1930*. Urbana: University of Illinois Press, 1994.

———. *Raising a Baby the Government Way: Mothers' Letters to the Children's Bureau*. New Brunswick, N.J.: Rutgers University Press, 1986.

Landry, Bart. *The New Black Middle Class*. Berkeley: University of California Press, 1987.

Leavitt, Judith Walzer. *Brought to Bed: Childbearing in America, 1750 to 1950*. New York: Oxford University Press, 1986.

——. *The Healthiest City: Milwaukee and the Politics of Health Reform*. Princeton, N.J.: Princeton University Press, 1982.

——, ed. *Women and Health in America: Historical Readings*. Madison: University of Wisconsin Press, 1984.

Leavitt, Judith Walzer and Ronald L. Numbers, eds. *Sickness and Health in America: Readings in the History of Medicine and Public Health*. Madison: University of Wisconsin Press, 1985.

Lerner, Gerda, ed. *Black Women in White America: A Documentary History*. New York: Random House, 1972.

——. *The Majority Finds Its Past: Placing Women in History*. New York: Oxford University Press, 1979.

Lightfoot, Sara Lawrence. *Balm in Gilead: Journey of a Healer*. Reading, Mass.: Addison-Wesley, 1988.

Litoff, Judy Barrett. *The American Midwife Debate: A Sourcebook on Its Modern Origins*. New York: Greenwood Press, 1986.

——. *American Midwives, 1860 to the Present*. Westport, Conn.: Greenwood Press, 1978.

Logan, Onnie Lee. *Motherwit: An Alabama Midwife's Story*. New York: E. P. Dutton, 1989.

Logan, Rayford W. and Michael R. Winston, eds. *Dictionary of American Negro Biography*. New York: W.W. Norton and Co., 1982.

McBride, David. *From TB to AIDS: Epidemics among Urban Blacks since 1900*. Albany: State University of New York Press, 1991.

——. *Integrating the City of Medicine: Blacks in Philadelphia Health Care, 1910–1965*. Philadelphia: Temple University Press, 1989.

McCarthy, Kathleen D. *Noblesse Oblige: Charity and Cultural Philanthropy in Chicago, 1849–1929*. Chicago: University of Chicago Press, 1982.

McMillen, Neil R. *Dark Journey: Black Mississippians in the Age of Jim Crow*. Urbana: University of Illinois Press, 1989.

McMurry, Linda O. *Recorder of the Black Experience: A Biography of Monroe Nathan Work*. Baton Rouge: Louisiana State University Press, 1985.

Mather, Frank Lincoln, ed. *Who's Who of the Colored Race: A General Biographical Dictionary of Men and Women of Colored Descent*. Chicago: F. L. Mather, 1915.

Meckel, Richard A. *Save the Babies: American Public Health Reform and the Prevention of Infant Mortality, 1850–1929*. Baltimore: Johns Hopkins University Press, 1990.

Meier, August. *Negro Thought in America, 1880–1915: Racial Ideologies in the Age of Booker T. Washington*. Ann Arbor: University of Michigan Press, 1963.

Melosh, Barbara. *"The Physician's Hand": Work, Culture and Conflict in American Nursing*. Philadelphia: Temple University Press, 1982.

Moldow, Gloria. *Women Doctors in Gilded-Age Washington: Race, Gender, and Professionalization*. Urbana: University of Illinois Press, 1987.

Morais, Herbert M. *The History of the Negro in Medicine*. New York: Publishers Company for the Association for the Study of Negro Life and History, 1967.

Morris, Aldon D. *The Origins of the Civil Rights Movement: Black Communities Organizing for Change*. New York: Free Press, 1984.

Moton, Robert R. *Finding a Way Out: An Autobiography*. Garden City, N.Y.: Doubleday, 1921.

Mott, Frederick D. and Milton I Roemer. *Rural Health and Medical Care*. New York: McGraw-Hill, 1948.

Mullan, Fitzhugh. *Plagues and Politics: The Story of the United States Public Health Service*. New York: Basic Books, 1989.

Muncy, Robyn. *Creating a Female Dominion in American Reform, 1890–1935*. New York: Oxford University Press, 1991.

Neverdon-Morton, Cynthia. *Afro-American Women of the South and the Advancement of the Race, 1895–1925*. Knoxville: University of Tennessee Press, 1989.

Newman, Debra. *Black History: A Guide to Civilian Records in the National Archives*. Washington, D.C.: National Archives Trust Fund Board, 1984.

Numbers, Ronald L. *Almost Persuaded: American Physicians and Compulsory Health Insurance, 1912–1920*. Baltimore: John Hopkins University Press, 1978.

Numbers, Ronald L. and Todd L. Savitt, eds. *Science and Medicine in the Old South*. Baton Rouge: Louisiana State University Press, 1989.

Parker, Marjorie H. *Alpha Kappa Alpha: 60 Years of Service*. n.p.: Alpha Kappa Sorority, 1966.

Pitrone, Jean Maddern. *Trailblazer: Negro Nurse in the American Red Cross*. New York: Harcourt Brace, 1969.

Poindexter, Hildrus. *My World of Reality*. Detroit: Balamp Publishing, 1973.

Rabinowitz, Howard N. *Race Relations in the Urban South, 1865–1890*. New York: Oxford University Press, 1978.

Rasmussen, Wayne D. and Gladys L. Baker. *The Department of Agriculture*. New York: Praeger, 1972.

Reverby, Susan M. *Ordered to Care: The Dilemma of American Nursing, 1850–1945*. Cambridge: Cambridge University Press, 1987.

Roe, Daphne A. *A Plague of Corn: The Social History of Pellagra*. Ithaca, N.Y.: Cornell University Press, 1973.

Rosen, George. *A History of Public Health*. New York: MD Publications, 1958.

Rosenkrantz, Barbara Gutmann. *Public Health and the State: Changing Views in Massachusetts, 1842–1936*. Cambridge, Mass.: Harvard University Press, 1972.

Rosner, David. *A Once Charitable Enterprise: Hospitals and Health Care in Brooklyn and New York, 1885–1915*. Cambridge: Cambridge University Press, 1982.

Ross, Edyth L. *Black Heritage in Social Welfare, 1860–1930*. Metuchen, N.J.: Scarecrow Press, 1978.

Rouse, Jacqueline Anne. *Lugenia Burns Hope: Black Southern Reformer*. Athens: University of Georgia Press, 1989.

Sacks, Karen Brodkin. *Caring by the Hour: Women, Work, and Organizing at Duke Medical Center*. Urbana: University of Illinois Press, 1988.

Salem, Dorothy. *To Better Our World: Black Women in Organized Reform, 1890–1920*. New York: Carlson Publishing, 1990.

Savitt, Todd L. *Medicine and Slavery: The Diseases and Health Care of Blacks in Antebellum Virginia*. Urbana: University of Illinois Press, 1978.

Scott, Anne Firor. *Natural Allies: Women's Associations in American History*. Urbana: University of Illinois Press, 1993.

Sewell, George Alexander and Margaret L. Dwight. *Mississippi Black History Makers*. Jackson: University Press of Mississippi, 1977, revised 1984.

Simonsen, Thordis, ed. *You May Plow Here: The Narrative of Sara Brooks*. New York: Touchtone Books, Simon and Schuster, 1986.

Sitkoff, Harvard. *A New Deal for Blacks: The Emergence of Civil Rights as a National Issue*. New York: Oxford University Press, 1978.

Spear, Allan H. *Black Chicago: The Making of a Negro Ghetto, 1890–1920*. Chicago: University of Chicago Press, 1967.

Starr, Paul. *The Social Transformation of American Medicine*. New York: Basic Books, 1982.

Staupers, Mabel Keaton. *No Time for Prejudice: The Story of the Integration of Negroes in Nursing in the United States*. New York: Macmillan, 1961.

Susie, Debra Anne. *In the Way of Our Grandmothers: A Cultural View of Twentieth-Century Midwifery in Florida*. Athens: University of Georgia Press, 1988.

Thoms, Adah B. *Pathfinders: A History of the Progress of Colored Graduate Nurses*. New York: Kay Printing House, 1929.

Tucker, Susan. *Telling Memories Among Southern Women: Domestic Workers and Their Employers in the Segregated South*. Baton Rouge: Louisiana State University Press, 1988.

Ulrich, Laurel Thatcher. *A Midwife's Tale: The Life of Martha Ballard, Based on Her Diary, 1785–1812*. New York: Knopf, 1990.

Underwood, Felix Joel and Richard Noble Whitfield. *Public Health and Medical Licensure in the State of Mississippi, 1938–1947*. Jackson, Miss.: Tucker Printing House, 1951.

Vogel, Morris J. *The Invention of the Modern Hospital, Boston, 1870–1930*. Chicago: University of Chicago Press, 1980.

Ware, Susan. *Beyond Suffrage: Women in the New Deal*. Cambridge, Mass.: Harvard University Press, 1981.

Washington, Booker T. *Up From Slavery: An Autobiography*. Association Press, 1901. Reprint New York: Lancer Books, 1968.

White, Evelyn C. *The Black Women's Health Book: Speaking for Ourselves*. Seattle, Wash.: Seal Press, 1990.

Williams, Patricia J. *The Alchemy of Race and Rights*. Cambridge, Mass.: Harvard University Press, 1991.

Williams, Ralph Chester. *The United States Public Health Service, 1798–1950*. Washington, D.C.: Commissioned Officers Association of the United States Public Health Service, 1951.

Wilson, Emily Herring. *Hope and Dignity: Older Black Women of the South*. Philadelphia: Temple University Press, 1983.

Wolters, Raymond. *Negroes and the Great Depression: The Problem of Economic Recovery*. Westport, Conn.: Greenwood Press, 1970.

Woodson, Carter Godwin. *The Negro Professional Man and the Community*. Washington, D.C.: Association for the Study of Negro Life and History, 1934.

ARTICLES

Aptheker, Bettina. "Woman Suffrage and the Crusade Against Lynching, 1890–1920." In Aptheker, *Woman's Legacy: Essays on Race, Sex, and Class*, 53–76. Amherst: University of Massachusetts Press, 1982.

Beardsley, Edward H. "Race as a Factor in Health." In *Women, Health and Medicine in America: A Historical Handbook*, ed. Rima D. Apple, 121–40. New York: Garland, 1990.

Berkeley, Kathleen C. "'Colored Ladies Also Contributed': Black Women's Activities from Benevolence to Social Welfare, 1866–1896." In *The Web of Southern Social Relations: Women, Family & Education*, ed. Walter J. Fraser, R. Frank Saunders, Jr., and Jon Wakelyn, 181–203. Athens: University of Georgia Press, 1985.

Brandt, Allan. "Racism and Research: The Case of the Tuskegee Syphilis Study." In *Sickness and Health in America: Readings in the History of Medicine and Public Health*, ed. Judith Walzer Leavitt and Ronald L. Numbers, 331–43. Madison: University of Wisconsin Press, 1984.

Breeden, James O. "Joseph Jones and Public Health in the New South." *Louisiana History* 32 (Fall 1991): 341–70.

Breen, William J. "Black Women and the Great War: Mobilization and Reform in the South." *Journal of Southern History* 44 (August 1978): 421–40.

Bridgforth, Lucie Robertson. "The Politics of Public Health Reform: Felix J. Underwood and the Mississippi State Board of Health, 1924–1958." *Public Historian* 6 (Summer 1984): 5–26.

Buhler-Wilkerson, Karen. "False Dawn: The Rise and Decline of Public Health Nursing in America, 1900–1930." In *Nursing History: New Perspectives, New Possibilities*, ed. Ellen Condliffe Lagemann, 89–106. New York: Teachers College Press, 1983.

Bushman, Richard L. and Claudia L. Bushman. "The Early History of Cleanliness in America." *Journal of American History* 74 (March 1988): 1213–38.

Cobb, James C. "'Somebody Done Nailed Us on the Cross': Federal Farm and Welfare Policy and the Civil Rights Movement in the Mississippi Delta." *Journal of American History* 77 (December 1990): 912–36.

Crosby, Earl W. "Limited Success Against Long Odds: The Black County Agent." *Agricultural History* 57 (July 1983): 277–88.

——. "The Struggle for Existence: The Institutionalization of the Black County Agent System." *Agricultural History* 60 (Spring 1986): 123–36.

Daniel, Pete. "Going among Strangers: Southern Reactions to World War II." *Journal of American History* 77 (December 1990): 886–911.

Dougherty, Molly C. "Southern Midwifery and Organized Health Care: Systems in Conflict." *Medical Anthropology: Cross Cultural Studies in Health and Illness* 6 (Spring 1982): 113–26.

Duffy, John. "Social Impact of Disease in Baltimore in the Twentieth Century." In *Sickness and Health in America: Readings in the History of Medicine and Public Health*, ed. Judith Walzer Leavitt and Ronald L. Numbers, 414–21. Madison: University of Wisconsin Press, 1985.

Fee, Elizabeth. "Sin vs. Science: Venereal Disease in Baltimore in the Twentieth Century." *Journal of the History of Medicine and Allied Sciences* 43 (April 1988): 141–64.

Ferguson, Earline Rae. "The Woman's Improvement Club of Indianapolis: Black Women Pioneers in Tuberculosis Work, 1903–1938." *Indiana Magazine of History* 84 (September 1988): 237–61.

Foster, Gaines M. "The Limitations of Federal Health Care for Freedmen, 1862–1868." *Journal of Southern History* 48 (August 1982): 349–72.

Galishoff, Stuart. "Germs Know No Color Line: Black Health and Public Policy in Atlanta, 1900–1918." *Journal of the History of Medicine and Allied Sciences* 40 (January 1985): 22–41.

Gamble, Vanessa Northington. "The Negro Hospital Renaissance: The Black Hospital Movement, 1920–1945." In *The American General Hospital: Communities and Social Contexts*, ed. Diana E. Long and Janet Golden, 82–105. Ithaca, N.Y.: Cornell University Press, 1989.

———. "The Provident Hospital Project: An Experiment in Race Relations and Medical Education." *Bulletin of the History of Medicine* 65 (Winter 1991): 457–75.

Gordon, Linda. "Black and White Visions of Welfare: Women's Welfare Activism, 1890–1945." *Journal of American History* 78 (September 1991): 559–90.

———. "Family Violence, Feminism, and Social Control." *Feminist Studies* 12 (Fall 1986): 453–78.

Hine, Darlene Clark. "The Ethel Johns Report: Black Women in the Nursing Profession, 1925." *Journal of Negro History* 67 (Fall 1982): 212–28.

———. "Lifting the Veil, Shattering the Silence: Black Women's History in Slavery and Freedom." In *The State of Afro-American History: Past, Present, and Future*, ed. Hine, 223–49. Baton Rouge: Louisiana State University Press, 1986.

———. "Mabel K. Staupers and the Integration of Black Nurses into the Armed Forces." In *Women and Health in America: Historical Readings*, ed. Judith Walzer Leavitt, 497–506. Madison: University of Wisconsin Press, 1984.

———. "Rape and the Inner Lives of Black Women in the Middle West: Preliminary Thoughts on the Culture of Dissemblance." *Signs: Journal of Women in Culture and Society* 14 (Summer 1989): 912–20.

———. " 'We Specialize in the Wholly Impossible': The Philanthropic Work of Black Women." In *Lady Bountiful Revisited: Women, Philanthropy, and Power*, ed. Kathleen D. McCarthy, 70–93. New Brunswick, N.J.: Rutgers University Press, 1990.

Holmes, Linda Janet. "African American Midwives in the South." In *The American Way of Birth*, ed. Pamela S. Eakins, 273–91. Philadelphia: Temple University Press, 1986.

Hoy, Suellen M. " 'Municipal Housekeeping': The Role of Women in Improving

Urban Sanitation Practices, 1880–1917." In *Pollution and Reform in American Cities, 1870–1930*, ed. Martin V. Melosi, 173–98. Austin: University of Texas Press, 1980.

Hunt, Marion. "Women and Childsaving: St. Louis Children's Hospital, 1879–1979." *Bulletin of the Missouri Historical Society* 36 (January 1980): 65–79.

James, Felix. "The Tuskegee Institute Movable School, 1906–1923." *Agricultural History* 45 (July 1971): 201–9.

Jefferson, Paul. "Working Notes on the Prehistory of Black Sociology: The Tuskegee Negro Conference." *Knowledge and Society: Studies in the Sociology of Culture Past and Present* 6 (1986): 119–51.

Jensen, Joan M. "Crossing Ethnic Barriers in the Southwest: Women's Agricultural Extension Education, 1914–1940." *Agricultural History* 60 (Spring 1986): 169–81.

Jones, Allen W. "The South's First Black Farm Agents." *Agricultural History* 50 (October 1976): 636–44.

———. "Thomas M. Campbell: Black Agricultural Leader of the New South." *Agricultural History* 53 (January 1979): 42–59.

Kaplan, Temma. "Female Consciousness and Collective Action: The Case of Barcelona, 1910–1918." *Signs: Journal of Women and Culture in Society* 7 (Spring 1982): 545–66.

Kobrin, Frances E. "The American Midwife Controversy: A Crisis of Professionalization." In *Sickness and Health in America: Readings in the History of Medicine and Public Health*, ed. Judith Walzer Leavitt and Ronald L. Numbers, 197–205. Madison: University of Wisconsin Press, 1985.

Krieger, Nancy. "Shades of Difference: Theoretical Underpinnings of the Medical Controversy on Black/White Differences in the United States, 1830–1870." *International Journal of Health Services* 17, 2 (1987): 259–78.

Ladd-Taylor, Molly. "'Grannies' and 'Spinsters': Midwife Education Under the Sheppard-Towner Act." *Journal of Social History* 22 (Winter 1988): 255–75.

———. "Women's Health and Public Policy." In *Women, Health, and Medicine in America: A Historical Handbook*, ed. Rima D. Apple, 391–410. New York: Garland, 1990.

Lawson, Steven F. "Freedom Then, Freedom Now: The Historiography of the Civil Rights Movement." *American Historical Review* 96 (April 1991): 456–71.

Leavitt, Judith Walzer. "Medicine in Context: A Review Essay of the History of Medicine." *American Historical Review* 95 (December 1990): 1471–84.

Levine, Lawrence W. "Marcus Garvey and the Politics of Revitalization." In *Black Leaders in the Twentieth Century*, ed. John Hope Franklin and August Meier, 105–38. Urbana: University of Illinois Press, 1982.

Litoff, Judy Barrett. "'Granny' Midwifery." In *Handbook of American Women's History*, ed. Angela Howard Zophy, 238. New York: Garland Publishing, 1990.

———. "Midwives and History." In *Women, Health, and Medicine in America: A Historical Handbook*, ed. Rima D. Apple, 443–58. New York: Garland, 1990.

Marable, Manning. "The Politics of Black Land Tenure, 1877–1915." *Agricultural History* 53 (January 1979): 142–52.

Morantz, Regina Markell. "Making Women Modern: Middle-Class Women and Health Reform in Nineteenth-Century America." In *Women and Health in America: Historical Readings*, ed. Judith Walzer Leavitt, 346–58. Madison: University of Wisconsin Press, 1984.

Numbers, Ronald L. "The Third Party: Health Insurance in America." In *Sickness and Health in America: Readings in the History of Medicine and Public Health*, ed. Judith Walzer Leavitt and Ronald L. Numbers, 233–47. Madison: University of Wisconsin Press, 1985.

Payne, Charles. "Men Led, But Women Organized: Movement Participation of Women in the Mississippi Delta." In *Women in the Civil Rights Movement*, ed. Vicki L. Crawford, Jacqueline Anne Rouse, and Barbara Woods, 1–11. New York: Carlson, 1990.

Pyle, Gerald F. "The Geography and Mortality of the 1918 Influenza Pandemic." *Bulletin of the History of Medicine* 65 (Spring 1991): 4–21.

Rodrique, Jessie M. "The Black Community and the Birth-Control Movement." In *Unequal Sisters: A Multicultural Reader in U.S. Women's History*, ed. Ellen Carol DuBois and Vicki L. Ruiz, 333–44. New York: Routledge, 1990.

Rosen, George. "The First Neighborhood Health Center Movement: Its Rise and Fall." In *Sickness and Health in America: Readings in the History of Medicine and Public Health*, ed. Judith Walzer Leavitt and Ronald L. Numbers, 475–89. Madison: University of Wisconsin Press, 1985.

Ross, B. Joyce. "Mary McLeod Bethune and the National Youth Administration: A Case Study of Power Relationships in the Black Cabinet of Franklin D. Roosevelt." In *Black Leaders of the Twentieth Century*, ed. John Hope Franklin and August Meier, 191–219. Urbana: University of Illinois Press, 1982.

Rudwick, Elliot. "The Niagara Movement." In *The Making of Black America: Essays in Negro Life and History*, ed. August Meier and Elliot Rudwick, 2: 131–48. New York: Atheneum, 1969.

Savitt, Todd L. "Entering A White Profession: Black Physicians in the New South." *Bulletin of the History of Medicine* 61 (Winter 1987): 507–40.

Schor, Joel. "The Black Presence in the U.S. Cooperative Extension Service Since 1945: An American Quest for Service and Equity." *Agricultural History* 60 (Spring 1986): 137–53.

Scott, Anne Firor. "Most Invisible of All: Black Women's Voluntary Associations." *Journal of Southern History* 56 (February 1990): 3–22.

Shaw, Stephanie J. "Black Club Women and the Creation of the National Association of Colored Women." *Journal of Women's History* 3 (Fall 1991): 10–25.

Shick, Tom W. "Race, Class and Medicine: 'Bad Blood' in Twentieth-Century America." *Journal of Ethnic Studies* 10 (Summer 1982): 97–105.

Torchia, Marion M. "The Tuberculosis Movement and the Race Question, 1890–1950." *Bulletin of the History of Medicine* 49 (Summer 1975): 152–68.

Walsh, Mary Roth. "Feminist Showplace." In *Women and Health in America: Historical Readings*, ed. Judith Walzer Leavitt, 392–405. Madison: University of Wisconsin Press, 1984.

Warner, John Harley. "The Idea of Southern Medical Distinctiveness: Medical

Knowledge and Practice in the Old South." In *Sickness and Health in America: Readings in the History of Medicine and Public Health*, ed. Judith Walzer Leavitt and Ronald L. Numbers, 53–70. Madison: University of Wisconsin Press, 1985.

White, Deborah Gray. "The Cost of Club Work, the Price of Black Feminism." In *Visible Women: New Essays on American Activism*, ed. by Nancy A. Hewitt and Suzanne Lebsock, 247–69. Urbana: University of Illinois Press, 1993.

White, E. Frances. "Africa on My Mind: Gender, Counter Discourse and African-American Nationalism." *Journal of Women's History* 2 (Spring 1990): 73–97.

——. "Listening to the Voices of Black Feminism." *Radical America* 18, 2–3 (1984): 7–25.

THESES AND UNPUBLISHED MANUSCRIPTS

Borst, Charlotte G. "Catching Babies: The Change From Midwife to Physician-Attended Childbirth in Wisconsin, 1870–1930." Ph.D. diss., University of Wisconsin, Madison, 1989.

Chappell, Edith P. and John F. Hume. "A Black Oasis: Tuskegee Institute's Fight Against Infantile Paralysis, 1941–1975." Unpublished manuscript, Tuskegee University, 1987, courtesy of Chappell.

Cooke, Michael Anthony. "The Health of Blacks During Reconstruction, 1862–1870." Ph.D. diss., University of Maryland, 1983.

Dickson, Lynda Faye. "The Early Club Movement Among Black Women in Denver, 1890–1925." Ph.D. diss., University of Colorado, Boulder, 1982.

Gamble, Vanessa Northington. "The Negro Hospital Renaissance: The Black Hospital Movement, 1920–1940." Ph.D. diss., University of Pennsylvania, 1987.

Hamilton, Tullia Kay Brown. "The National Association of Colored Women, 1896–1920." Ph.D. diss., Emory University, 1978.

Jackson, James Willis. "The Search for Something Better: Ida Louise Jackson's Life Story." Unpublished manuscript, no date, courtesy of Jackson.

Legan, Marshall Scott. "The Evolution of Public Health Services in Mississippi, 1865–1910." Ph.D. diss., University of Mississippi, 1968.

May, Jude Thomas. "The Medical Care of Blacks in Louisiana During the Occupation and Reconstruction, 1862–1868: Its Social and Political Background." Ph.D. diss., Tulane University, 1971.

Mayer, John. "Private Charities in Chicago from 1871 to 1915." Ph.D. diss., University of Minnesota, 1978.

Reagan, Leslie J. "When Abortion Was a Crime: The Legal and Medical Regulation of Abortion, Chicago, 1880–1973." Ph.D. diss., University of Madison-Wisconsin, 1991.

Schwalm, Leslie. "The Meaning of Freedom: African-American Women and Their Transition from Slavery to Freedom in Lowcountry South Carolina." Ph.D. diss., University of Wisconsin-Madison, 1991.

Sloan, Patricia Ellen. "A History of the Establishment and Early Development of

Selected Schools of Nursing for Afro-Americans, 1886–1906." Ph.D. diss., Teachers College, Columbia University, 1978.

Tillman, Elvena Bage. "The Rights of Childhood: The National Child Welfare Movement, 1890–1919." Ph.D. diss., University of Wisconsin-Madison, 1968.

Warner, Margaret Ellen. "Public Health in the New South: Government, Medicine and Society in the Control of Yellow Fever." Ph.D. diss., Harvard University, 1983.

Index

University of Pennsylvania Press
Studies in Health, Illness, and Caregiving
Joan E. Lynaugh, General Editor

Barbara Bates. *Bargaining for Life: A Social History of Tuberculosis, 1876–1938.* 1992.

Michael D. Calabria and Janet A. Macrae, editors. Suggestions for Thought *by Florence Nightingale: Selections and Commentaries.* 1993.

Janet Golden and Charles Rosenberg. *Pictures of Health: A Photographic History of Health Care in Philadelphia.* 1991.

Anne Hudson Jones, ed. *Images of Nurses: Perspectives from History, Art, and Literature.* 1987.

June S. Lowenberg. *Caring and Responsibility: The Crossroads Between Holistic Practice and Traditional Medicine.* 1989.

Peggy McGarrahan. *Transformation and Transcendence: Caring for HIV Patients in New York City.* 1993.

Elizabeth Norman. *Women at War: The Story of Fifty Military Nurses Who Served in Vietnam.* 1990.

Bonnie Blair O'Connor. *Healing Traditions: Alternative Medicine and the Health Professions.* 1995.

Anne Opie. *There's Nobody There: Community Care of Confused Older People.* 1992.

Elizabeth Brown Pryor. *Clara Barton, Professional Angel.* 1987.

Margarete Sandelowski. *With Child in Mind: Studies of the Personal Encounter with Infertility.* 1993.

Susan L. Smith. *Sick and Tired of Being Sick and Tired: Black Women's Health Activism in America, 1890–1950.* 1995.

Nancy Tomes. *The Art of Asylum-Keeping: Thomas Story Kirkbride and the Origins of American Psychiatry.* 1994.

Zane Robinson Wolf. *Nurses' Work, The Sacred and The Profane.* 1988.

Jacqueline Zalumas. *Caring in Crisis: An Oral History of Critical Care Nursing.* 1994.